Drugs Easily Explained

Roland Seifert

Drugs Easily Explained

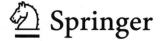 Springer

Roland Seifert
Institute of Pharmacology, Hannover Medical School
Hannover, Germany

ISBN 978-3-031-12187-6   ISBN 978-3-031-12188-3   (eBook)
https://doi.org/10.1007/978-3-031-12188-3

Cover image: Felipe Caparrós/stock.adobe.com

This Springer imprint is published by the registered company Springer Nature Switzerland AG.
The registered company address is: Gewerbestrasse 11, 6330 Cham, Switzerland

Preface

Billions of people worldwide take drugs daily to treat important diseases. However, in many cases, neither the doctor nor the pharmacist takes the time to explain to the patient why a certain drug should be taken, how the drug works, and what adverse reactions to expect. Of course, on the Internet, the patient can find "everything" on any given drug. But how reliable and understandable is this information? Moreover, most internet resources fail to point out connections between various diseases and drug interactions. This book provides an overview of the most common diseases and the drugs used for their treatment. The book has been designed for a general audience. The book provides patients with essential information on how drugs work and what adverse effects and drug interactions can be expected. Finally, the book provides patients with advice on what can be done from their side to improve drug therapy and safety. Summaries, memos, tables, and schemes support the information process. This book is an adaptation, for an international audience, of the book *Medikamente leicht erklärt* (2021) [ISBN: 978-3-662-62329-9].

I would like to thank Mrs. Annette Stanke for her expert support with the translation of the book. I also thank Mrs. Susanne Dathe from Springer Nature for her support to realize this book.

Hannover, Germany
October 2022

Roland Seifert

Contents

Abbreviations

5-ARI	5-alpha reductase inhibitor
ACE	angiotensin-converting enzyme
ADHD	attention deficit–hyperactivity disorder
ADP	adenosine diphosphate (an inflammatory molecule leading to platelet clumping)
ADR	adverse drug reaction
ARB	angiotensin receptor blocker
ASA	acetylsalicylic acid
cGMP	cyclic guanosine monophosphate
CHD	coronary heart disease
COMT	catechol-*O*-methyltransferase
COPD	chronic obstructive pulmonary disease
COVID-19	coronavirus disease 2019
COX	cyclooxygenase
DMARD	disease-modifying antirheumatic drug
DNA	deoxyribonucleic acid (hereditary material in humans and in many pathogens of infectious diseases)
DOAC	direct oral anticoagulant (also called NOAC [new oral anticoagulant])
DPP4	dipeptidyl peptidase 4
ECG	electrocardiogram
ED	erectile dysfunction
EGF	epidermal growth factor
EMA	European Medicines Agency
EPI	epinephrine (also called adrenaline)
EPS	extrapyramidal symptom

g	gram (a unit of mass in which some drug dosages are measured; one gram [1 g] is equal to one thousand milligrams [1000 mg])
GABA	gamma-aminobutyric acid
G-CSF	granulocyte colony–stimulating factor
GERD	gastroesophageal reflux disease
GLP-1	glucagon-like peptide 1
GTN	glyceryl trinitrate
HbA_{1C}	hemoglobin A_{1c}
HER2	human epidermal growth factor receptor 2
H_1 receptor	histamine H_1 receptor
H_2 receptor	histamine H_2 receptor
HDL cholesterol	high-density lipoprotein cholesterol ("good" cholesterol)
HER2	human epidermal growth factor receptor 2
HMG-CoA	3-hydroxy-3-methylglutaryl coenzyme A
HRT	hormone replacement therapy (also known as menopausal hormone therapy [MHT])
ICS	inhaled corticosteroid (glucocorticoid)
IL	interleukin
INN	international nonproprietary name
INR	international normalized ratio (important in therapy with vitamin K antagonists)
IU	international unit
IU/kg	international units per kilogram
IU/mL	international units per milliliter
kg	kilogram
L	liter
LABA	long-acting beta receptor agonist
LAMA	long-acting muscarinic receptor antagonist
LDL cholesterol	low-density lipoprotein cholesterol ("bad" cholesterol)
LTRA	leukotriene receptor antagonist
MAO	monoamine oxidase
MCP	metoclopramide
MCRA	mineralocorticoid receptor antagonist
MDMA	3,4-methylenedioxy-methamphetamine (a psychotropic drug, also known as ecstasy)
mg	milligram (a unit of mass in which many drug dosages are measured; one gram [1 g] is equal to one thousand milligrams [1000 mg])
mg/dL	milligrams per deciliter
mGPCR	multiple G-protein-coupled receptor

MHT	menopausal hormone therapy (also known as hormone replacement therapy [HRT])
mL	milliliter
mmHg	millimeters of mercury (a unit in which blood pressure is measured)
mmol/L	millimoles per liter
MPH	methylphenidate
MRSA	multidrug-resistant *Staphylococcus aureus*
MTX	methotrexate
NO	nitric oxide
NOAC	new oral anticoagulant (also called DOAC [direct oral anticoagulant])
NSAID	nonsteroidal anti-inflammatory drug
NSMRI	nonselective monoamine reuptake inhibitor
PDE	phosphodiesterase
PGE	prostaglandin E
PPAR	peroxisome proliferator–activated receptor
PPI	proton pump inhibitor
PUD	peptic ulcer disease
RAAS	renin–angiotensin–aldosterone system
RANKL	receptor activator of nuclear factor kappa B ligand
RNA	ribonucleic acid (important for formation of proteins in humans and in many pathogens of infectious diseases; also hereditary material in many viruses)
SABA	short-acting beta receptor agonist
SAMA	short-acting muscarinic receptor antagonist
SARS-CoV-2	severe acute respiratory syndrome coronavirus 2
SERM	selective estrogen receptor modulator
SGLT2	sodium/glucose cotransporter 2
SSNRI	selective serotonin/noradrenaline reuptake inhibitor
SSRI	selective serotonin reuptake inhibitor
T3	thyronine
T4	thyroxine (an endogenous thyroid hormone; synthetic T4 is called levothyroxine)
TCA	tricyclic antidepressant
TDM	therapeutic drug monitoring (monitoring of drug concentrations in the blood)
TNF	tumor necrosis factor
TNM	Tumor–Node–Metastasis
TSH	thyroid-stimulating hormone
UV	ultraviolet

VEGF	vascular endothelial growth factor
WHO	World Health Organization
Z drugs	drugs (the prototype drug is zolpidem) with effects similar to those of benzodiazepines, only shorter and weaker
μg	microgram (a unit of mass in which only a few drug dosages are measured; one gram [1 g] is equal to one million micrograms [1,000,000 μg]; one milligram [1 mg] is equal to one thousand micrograms [1000 μg])

1

What Should I Know About Drugs?

Abstract This chapter is the basis for understanding all other chapters in this book. Therefore, you should read this chapter first. You will learn important medical concepts, such as the difference between a drug and a poison, and how to distinguish between a brand-name and a generic name. You will learn how homeopathic drugs work. The chapter gives you an overview of how drug development works. An important aspect is repurposing of known drugs for new areas of application. This is why many traditional drug class names no longer fit their current applications. For all readers who want to understand how drugs work in the body, one section explains the main drug targets. These are receptors, enzymes, channels, pumps, and the cell nucleus. Finally, the chapter discusses how drugs move through the body and what you need to know if you take many drugs.

1.1 Some Important Terms

Summary

Drugs have beneficial effects in the human body; poisons have harmful effects. Depending on the type of administration and the dose, a drug can become a poison, and vice versa. Even drugs without a pharmacologically active substance can produce effects. Such drugs are called placebos. However, placebos can cause adverse drug reactions (ADRs). This is called a nocebo effect. All drugs should be dosed with particular care in elderly people and children.

Memo

- Drugs have beneficial effects on humans.
- Drugs are assigned international nonproprietary names (INNs).
- The INN of a drug is understood worldwide.
- Poisons have harmful effects on humans.
- Drugs are marketed under brand-names or as generics under their INNs.
- Prescription and nonprescription drugs can cause ADRs.
- Homeopathic drugs work through a placebo effect.
- Placebos can have harmful effects (nocebo effects).
- Elderly people are particularly susceptible to ADRs and drug interactions.

Drugs Are Useful; Poisons Are Harmful

Figure 1.1 shows an overview of important terms related to drug therapy. The term "pharmacologically active substance" is superordinate and value neutral: an active substance is a chemical substance that can change bodily functions. This does not imply anything about the usefulness or harmfulness of its effect.

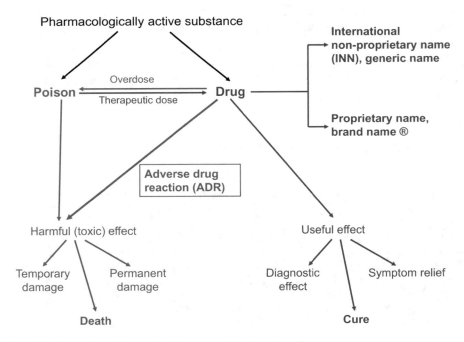

Fig. 1.1 Overview of important terms related to drug therapy

Drugs are pharmacologically active substances with beneficial effects on the human organism. At best, the beneficial effect entails curing the disease—for example, treating a bacterial infection with an antibacterial drug (antibiotic) that kills the causative pathogen (see Sect. 11.3). In many cases, however, a disease cannot be cured; only its symptoms are treated. Examples include pain therapy (see Chap. 2) and treatments for mental disorders (see Chap. 9). Substances used in diagnosis of diseases also belong to the category of drugs. Contrast agents for magnetic resonance imaging are a particularly important example. In addition, a drug can cause an ADR in therapeutically effective doses. Instead of the term "ADR", the term "side effects" is often used, but the former is more accurate. In this book, the term "ADR" is used.

Poisons are pharmacologically active substances with harmful (toxic) effects on the human organism. Determining whether a pharmacologically active substance is a drug or a poison is not trivial. If a patient takes a drug in an overdose by mistake or with suicidal intent, it can become a poison. As examples, opioid analgesics (e.g., morphine, derived from opium from the opium poppy), which are used for severe pain in cancer therapy, can lead to respiratory arrest (cessation of breathing) in an overdose (see Sect. 2.2), and vitamin K antagonists (the prototype drug is warfarin), which are used to treat heart attacks and strokes, can cause severe bleeding if overdosed (see Sect. 5.2).

The poison of the deadly nightshade (atropine) can cause intoxication if the fruit is consumed accidentally, but when used in the eye, atropine can be used to treat inflammation of the iris. If one consumes canned food contaminated by the bacterium *Clostridium botulinum*, the botulinum neurotoxin (Botox) can cause respiratory arrest. If, on the other hand, botulinum neurotoxin is injected specifically into cramped (dystonic) muscles (e.g., for treatment of torticollis), it can lead to therapeutically desired muscle relaxation.

The question whether a pharmacologically active substance acts as a drug or as a poison depends on the dose and the application. An overdose of any drug can make it act as a poison. However, not every poison acts as a drug when used in a lower dose.

A drug as such is not used in its undiluted form in humans; instead, it is "packaged" with various pharmaceutical excipients. The excipients bring the drug into solution, shield it during gastric passage, or fill tablets. Such preparations facilitate or delay absorption of drugs into the body in a manner appropriate to the treatment (see Sect. 1.5).

A drug is marketed under a brand-name or under its INN as a generic. A brand-name is recognizable by the "®" symbol, standing for "registered trademark". Naming of drugs is so important for the patient that it is dealt with in a separate section of this chapter (see Sect. 1.2).

Drugs are mostly produced by pharmaceutical companies and less often in pharmacies. The main task of pharmacies is to dispense drugs and to provide drug advice. Internet pharmacies are becoming more widespread. Although Internet shopping is more convenient, the important aspect of personal advice is lost.

A distinction is made between prescription drugs, which can only be dispensed on a doctor's prescription, and nonprescription drugs, which can be obtained without a doctor's prescription. The prescription/nonprescription status of drugs differs between countries, reflecting cultural differences.

It is a common misconception that only prescription drugs cause ADRs and that nonprescription drugs are safe and do not cause ADRs. For example, some nonprescription painkillers such as paracetamol (acetaminophen) can cause liver damage (see Sect. 2.1). Ibuprofen can cause severe kidney damage and high blood pressure (see Sects. 2.1 and 5.1). Antihistamines in overdose can cause symptoms similar to those of poisoning with the fruit of the deadly nightshade plant (antimuscarinic syndrome; see Sect. 4.1). These examples show how important it is for you to take personal responsibility for correct use of drugs.

An Overview of Different Dosage Forms

Commonly used dosage forms of drugs are tablets, capsules, and drops, all of which are suitable for oral administration (PO). Different solutions are formulated for administration under the skin (subcutaneous [SC]), into a muscle (intramuscular [IM]) or into a vein (intravenous [IV]). An example of a subcutaneously administered drug is an insulin preparation used for treatment of type 1 diabetes (see Sect. 6.1). Self-injection of epinephrine (adrenaline) with an epinephrine auto-injector is an example of an intramuscular injection (see Sect. 4.1). In some cases, drugs that are intended to exert systemic effects are supplied as skin patches or as rectal suppositories. For skin diseases, a variety of ointments, creams, and lotions (preparations with lower fat content) are available.

What Is a Placebo Effect?

Even a drug without a pharmacologically active substance can show beneficial effects. These drugs are called placebos. How does a placebo work? Prescribing, dispensing, and taking a drug is a complex process. The advice and attention given by the doctor and pharmacist and the patient's expectations play important roles. Placebos are therefore particularly effective in areas of application where psychological factors have a major influence (e.g., headaches, insomnia, gastrointestinal disorders, pain [see Sects. 2.1 and 2.2], and depressive moods [see Sect. 9.2]).

The placebo effect is so important that in clinical trials in which drugs are tested for their efficacy prior to approval, a placebo group is included whenever possible and ethically justifiable—except, for example, in the case of cancer (see Sect. 11.1). Only if a new drug shows a better effect than a placebo will it be approved.

It is often difficult to distinguish whether the effect of a drug is due to the pharmacologically active substance or whether a placebo effect accounts for it. Genuine placebos are (so far) hardly ever prescribed, although conscious prescribing of a placebo for a patient (i.e., the patient knows it is a placebo) can cause therapeutic effects.

Homeopathic drugs are popular with many patients. This is because homeopathy takes a holistic approach to diseases. Patients appreciate holism. Homeopathic drugs contain pharmacologically active substances in very high dilutions so that, according to scientific laws, no pharmacological effect can take place. If highly diluted ("high-potency") homeopathic drugs "work", this is again a placebo effect based on attention, expectation, and selective observation and perception.

What Is a Nocebo Effect?

Placebos can cause ADRs. The suggestive power of the doctor and pharmacist and the patient's expectations play important roles. Frequently observed nocebo effects are fatigue, headache, and gastrointestinal complaints. If a placebo shows an ADR, we speak of a nocebo effect. Consequently, homeopathic drugs show nocebo effects as well.

Do Drugs Work the Same for Everyone?

No, they don't. The effect of a drug depends on the patient's age. Newborns, infants, children, and elderly people react differently from adults. Elderly people are particularly susceptible to ADRs. Therefore, they should take as few drugs as possible. The data on use of drugs in pregnancy are, in many cases, unsatisfactory and incomplete. Therefore, if therapy is required in pregnancy, well-tried drugs should be preferred. Sex, ethnicity, dietary habits, alcohol consumption, and cigarette consumption can influence the efficacy of drugs.

Drugs from completely different areas of application can influence each other in their effects. The best way to avoid such interactions is to use as few different drugs as possible. Polypharmacy is a huge problem these days because many people suffer from numerous diseases.

1.2   Drug Names

Summary

Many drug names seem like a foreign language. But there are a few tricks to help you find your way around. The most important information on a drug package is the INN of the drug. In many cases, a drug class–specific word stem in an INN provides information about the class to which that drug belongs. Brand-names are often suggestive. Historically developed names of drug classes are often problematic against the background of significantly increased knowledge and changed drug use in recent years.

Memo

- Many drug classes can be recognized by word stems in the drug names.
- Several older drug names have no drug-specific word stems, unfortunately.
- The naming of biologicals—drugs (mainly proteins) that are produced biotechnologically)—presents a major language barrier.
- Brand-names often have a suggestive character.
- Preference should be given to the INN.
- Most diseases can be treated well with generic drugs.
- Supply bottlenecks affecting supply of generics are becoming increasingly frequent because of centralized production.
- Many traditional drug class names are misleading.
- Drug classes should be named in accordance with their mechanisms of action.

Are Drug Names Just Medical Jargon?

Countless drugs are on the market. It is impossible for doctors, pharmacists, and patients to keep track of them all. To make matters worse, many drug names are difficult to pronounce. Of course, many people have heard of Aspirin®, Viagra®, and Ritalin®, but what about tongue twisters such as ustekinumab, aflibercept, or pembrolizumab? These drug names are difficult to remember and difficult to pronounce.

The purpose of this section is to show you that the names of frequently prescribed drugs contain drug-specific word stems that tell you something about the drug classes and the mechanisms of action. By correctly deciphering the INN of a drug, you can obtain important information about its indications and about similarly acting drugs.

Several drug classes, and thus their indications, can be recognized by characteristic word stems in the INNs of the respective drugs. Table 1.1 shows, in alphabetical order, some frequently prescribed drugs (in column 1), the drug classes (in column 2), and the characteristic word stems that all drug names in each class contain (in column 3). In most cases, the word stem is a suffix; more rarely, it is a prefix or is in the middle of the name.

All beta blocker names have the suffix "_olol" (see Sect. 5.1). The most important lipid-lowering drug names are identified by the suffix "_statin", which is why this drug class is referred to as statins. The names of angiotensin-converting enzyme (ACE) inhibitors commonly used for treatment of cardiovascular diseases have the suffix "_pril" (see Sects. 5.1–5.3). The names of angiotensin receptor blockers (ARBs, angiotensin receptor antagonists) have the suffix "_sartan" and are therefore known as sartans (see Sects. 5.1–5.3). The names of serotonin-3 receptor antagonists end in "_setron", from which the name setrons derives (see Sect. 11.1). Finally, the triptans are serotonin-1 receptor agonists with the suffix "_triptan" in their names (see Sect. 2.1).

Drugs whose names have a common suffix have similar mechanisms of action. Therefore, it is often possible to switch between different drugs in the same class that have a common suffix in their names without significantly changing the treatment. This process is referred to as substitution.

The names of benzodiazepines, which can cause addiction (see Sect. 8.2), can have either of two suffixes: "_zolam" for short-acting drugs and "_zepam" for long-acting drugs. In the case of the antibiotically active cephalosporins, the drug-specific word stem "cef_" is at the beginning of the drug name. In the case of factor Xa inhibitors, the drug-specific word stem "_xa_" is hidden in the middle of the drug name. These drugs are known as xabans.

Table 1.1 Recognition of important drug names by their characteristic word stems

Drug	Drug class	Drug-specific word stem in drug name
Alendronate	Bisphosphonates	_dronate
Amlodipine	Calcium channel blockers (calcium antagonists)	_dipine
Amoxicillin	Penicillins	_cillin
Candesartan	Angiotensin receptor blockers (ARBs, sartans)	_sartan
Cefaclor	Cephalosporins	Cef_
Ciprofloxacin	Fluoroquinolones	_floxacin
Clonidine	Alpha-2 receptor agonists	_nidine
Clopidogrel	Adenosine diphosphate (ADP) receptor antagonists	_grel
Clotrimazole	Azole antimycotics (azoles)	_azole
Diazepam	Long-acting benzodiazepines	_zepam
Empagliflozin	Sodium glucose cotransporter 2 (SGLT2) inhibitors (gliflozins)	_gliflozin
Formoterol	Beta receptor agonists (beta sympathomimetics)	_terol
Furosemide	Loop diuretics	_semide
Metoprolol	Beta receptor antagonists (beta blockers)	_olol
Midazolam	Short-acting benzodiazepines	_zolam
Montelukast	Leukotriene receptor antagonists (LTRAs, lukasts)	_lukast
Ondansetron	Serotonin-3 receptor antagonists (setrons)	_setron
Pantoprazole	Proton pump inhibitors (PPIs)	_prazole
Ramipril	Angiotensin-converting enzyme (ACE) inhibitors	_pril
Rivaroxaban	Factor Xa inhibitors (xabans; direct oral anticoagulants [DOACs], new oral anticoagulants [NOACs])	_xa_
Roflumilast	Phosphodiesterase type 4 (PDE4) inhibitors	_last
Sildenafil	Phosphodiesterase type 5 (PDE5) inhibitors	_afil
Simvastatin	Lipid-lowering drugs (statins)	_statin
Sitagliptin	Dipeptidyl peptidase-4 (DPP4) inhibitors (gliptins)	_gliptin
Sumatriptan	Serotonin-1 receptor agonists (triptans)	_triptan
Xylometazoline	Alpha-1 receptor agonists	_zoline

In the tables in this book, drug-specific word stems are shown in bold text. In the case of factor Xa inhibitors, the presence of several colloquial names often leads to misunderstandings. For many drugs (especially for drugs introduced many years ago), unfortunately, *no* drug-specific word stems exist. The only way to help here is to look them up in books and on the Internet. Examples of such drugs are cetirizine, clemastine, clozapine, diphenhydramine, metamizole (dipyrone), metformin, paracetamol (acetaminophen), sertraline, tramadol, and valproic acid. It is easy to confuse the word stems "_lukast" and "_last". Drug class abbreviations with generic name word stems are formed only where this is linguistically possible

ACE angiotensin-converting enzyme, *ADP* adenosine diphosphate, *ARB* angiotensin receptor blocker, *DOAC* direct oral anticoagulant, *DPP4* dipeptidyl peptidase-4, *LTRA* leukotriene receptor antagonist, *NOAC* new oral anticoagulant, *PDE4* phosphodiesterase type 4, *PDE5* phosphodiesterase type 5, *PPI* proton pump inhibitor, *SGLT2* sodium glucose cotransporter 2

Biologicals are drugs (mainly proteins) that are produced biotechnologically. These include specific antibodies (see Sects. 4.1, 6.3, 10.2, 11.1, and 11.3). Although the suffix "_ab" indicates that the drug is an antibody, the names of these drugs often say little about their mechanism of action and clinical use. The names of many biologicals are difficult to pronounce. This makes communication between the doctor, pharmacist, and patient difficult. As more biologicals are approved, an immense communication problem is building up.

Perhaps the complicated INNs of biologicals are deliberately intended to conceal the mechanism of action and thus the interchangeability of the biological with a biosimilar (a generic drug that is highly similar to a previously approved proprietary biological) for commercial reasons, because this makes it easier to bind a doctor to a particular biological in prescribing and makes substitution more difficult.

Names of Old Drugs

We have valuable drugs whose mechanisms of action were not yet known when they were developed. These drugs have INNs from which no useful information about the mechanism of action or the indications can be derived. These drug names must be looked up to find out to which drug class they belong. Examples of such drugs are the analgesics paracetamol (acetaminophen) and metamizole (dipyrone; see Sect. 2.1), the antihistamine clemastine (see Sect. 4.1), the antidiabetic metformin (see Sect. 6.1), and the antiepileptic valproic acid (see Sect. 8.2).

Problems Associated with Use of Brand-Names

If a pharmaceutical company brings a new drug onto the market, this drug enjoys patent protection for several (usually 10) years. The company brings it onto the market under a brand-name (with a registered trademark, "®") and then has a monopoly for this drug during this period and can charge high prices. The prices are justified by the companies with the argument that the development costs must be refinanced. Regrettably, there have been cases in which the profit motive was dominant.

In contrast to INNs, which often provide important information on the mechanism of action, brand-names are mostly fantasy names without reference to the mechanisms of action of the drugs. The lack of reference to the mechanisms of action in brand-names increases the risk of unintentional multiple prescriptions of drugs from the same drug class and nonrecognition of drug interactions.

Instead, brand-names often have a suggestive character and are intended to draw attention to the positive properties of the drugs. In the case of a brand-name drug, it is essential to pay attention to the INN, which is usually visible only in small print on the package. But the INN is much more important than the brand-name for assessing the mechanism of action, indications for use, and ADRs.

The name Acomplia® promised a complication-free and effective treatment for diabetes and obesity, but this drug was withdrawn from the market because of increased suicide rates and depression. The name Bonviva® promises a good life without drawing attention to the fact that use of bisphosphonates in osteoporosis can cause severe ADRs, such as jaw damage (see Sect. 6.3). The name Champix® has several possible associations: the drug is a "champion" in nicotine withdrawal (i.e., it is particularly effective), and you will feel as good as after a glass of champagne. The reality is different. Varenicline, which is contained in Champix®, is not effective in nicotine withdrawal, nor do patients feel well. As a final example, the name Halcion® promises happiness without pointing out that addiction and withdrawal symptoms may occur (see Sect. 8.2).

The Difference Between a Brand-Name Drug and a Generic Drug

Once the patent for a brand-name drug has expired, other manufacturers can bring the drug onto the market. However, they can launch this drug only as generic, which is sold under the INN. Therefore, the INN of the drug is printed in correspondingly large letters on the packaging. As soon as a generic drug is launched onto the market, prices fall because of competition. As a result, the drug sold under a brand-name becomes less expensive. Generic manufacturers undercut the prices of drugs sold under brand-names.

If your doctor switches you from an expensive brand-name drug to an inexpensive generic drug, you may suspect that you are now being treated "worse" than before. However, this is usually not the case, because the generic manufacturer must prove that their drug is no different from the brand-name drug in terms of pharmaceutical quality and efficacy. A switch from a brand-name drug to a generic drug is usually possible without a decrease in the quality of therapy. Occasionally, however, a switch between two different formulations of the same drug can result in new ADRs caused not by the pharmacologically active substance itself (which is the same in both formulations) but by differences in the excipients that the different formulations contain.

If you take a generic drug, every doctor and pharmacist in the world knows which drug it is. This is of importance in a globalized world and simplifies drug therapy during travel. Brand-names, on the other hand, are often country specific. If you take a drug with a brand-name, the doctor or pharmacist may have to do some research, and there will be some uncertainty. So, overall, there are many reasons to prescribe generics when possible.

Meanwhile, more biologicals are losing their patent protection. Generic biologicals are called biosimilars. Inexpensive biosimilars have efficacy comparable to that of the much more expensive biologicals, although this is denied by the manufacturers of the biologicals. Use of biosimilars offers large savings opportunities for health care systems.

Problems Associated with Use of Generics

Widespread use of generic drugs can bring about large cost savings in health care systems. This is in the interests of all insured persons, so that financial collapse of health care systems in aging societies does not occur. The sad downside, however, is that production of generic drugs is becoming extremely centralized. Often, only one production site worldwide remains. If something goes wrong there, or if supply chains are interrupted (as in the COVID 19 pandemic), worldwide problems in the supply of important drugs emerge. Such problems have occurred repeatedly—for example, with ibuprofen (see Sect. 2.1), opioid analgesics (see Sect. 2.2), acetylsalicylic acid (see Sect. 5.2), thyroid hormones (see Sect. 6.2), and certain antibiotics (see Sect. 11.3).

Another problem is that because of cost pressure, production of drugs has been increasingly "optimized". This has led to contamination of certain drugs with carcinogenic substances (see Sect. 11.1). Current examples include the ARB valsartan (see Sects. 5.1–5.3) and the histamine H_2 receptor blocker ranitidine (see Sects. 3.1 and 3.2). Such impurities lead to recall of drugs and to uncertainty among patients.

In such increasingly frequent supply shortages, your doctor and your pharmacist must try to pick out alternative drugs for you, which is often a challenge. For these reasons, "standard" drugs should be produced regionally, and drug reserves should be available in every country. Considering that it is possible to treat many common diseases with the approximately 100 drugs described in this book, this is not too ambitious a goal.

Problems Associated with Traditional Drug Class Names

Many of the drugs used today were developed decades ago. Often, it was not known (and in some cases, it is still not known) how these drugs work. It was known only that they had therapeutic effects in certain diseases. Accordingly, drug classes used to be named in accordance with their indications. Generations of doctors and pharmacists, and thus patients, learned this system. In the meantime, however, knowledge about the mechanisms of action of many drugs has improved and many indications have changed. Therefore, old drug class terms do not fit the indications anymore.

In the long term, the traditional terms will be replaced by modern terms. This poses a big practical problem: young doctors and pharmacists learn the new terms in college but must know the old terms to be able to communicate with older colleagues and patients. In this book—out of consideration for most doctors, pharmacists, and patients—the traditional terms are used, but the modern terms are additionally introduced. Modern nomenclature of drug classes will increase drug safety and reduce the incidence of ADRs. Above all, this is in your best interests as a patient. A glossary at the end of the book serves as an explanation for some medical terms.

Although replacement of traditional drug class names by modern names will be tedious, the effort is worthwhile. It makes it easier to understand how drugs work and which drug is to be used for a certain disease. By reading this book, you can participate in and contribute to improvements in drug therapy.

The two examples given below are used to illustrate problems associated with traditional drug class names.

Example 1: Antidepressants
The importance of changing the names of drug classes is particularly obvious for drugs used for mental disorders (see Chap. 9). Every patient knows the term "antidepressants". Originally, this drug class was developed for treatment of depression, hence the term "antidepressants". In the meantime, however, antidepressants have been successfully introduced for a variety of other disorders that have nothing to do with depression. These include cancer pain (see Sect. 11.1), pain in polyneuropathies (see Sect. 2.1), and migraines, as well as anxiety and panic disorders (see Sect. 9.2). It is therefore a challenge for the doctor to explain to the patient why they are being prescribed an antidepressant although they are not depressed. Since depression remains a stigmatized disorder, the patient may suspect they do in fact have depression, which is merely being renamed. As a result, the patient looks for depression symptoms in

(continued)

(continued)

themselves and may find them, or they do not take their antidepressant because they are not depressed, which in turn results in their condition not improving. Therefore, antidepressants are better referred to as "norepinephrine/serotonin enhancers" in modern medical nomenclature, in accordance with their mode of action. This term avoids stigmatization of the patient as being "depressed" and facilitates easier application of these drugs in different diseases.

Example 2: Nonsteroidal Anti-inflammatory Drugs

Another example of problematic drug naming is the nonsteroidal anti-inflammatory (antirheumatic) drugs (NSAIDs). In the 1950s, it was discovered that "steroids" or "cortisone" (more precisely, glucocorticoids) could be used to treat rheumatoid arthritis effectively (see Sect. 11.2). For this reason, glucocorticoids were called steroidal anti-inflammatory drugs. However, it soon became apparent that they could cause severe ADRs in long-term use. Therefore, alternatives were sought and NSAIDs were developed. The term "NSAID" suggests efficacy similar to that of steroidal drugs with significantly reduced ADRs in long-term use. Although it emerged that NSAIDs can cause kidney problems, gastrointestinal ulcers, and high blood pressure (see Sects. 3.2 and 5.1) with long-term use, the term "NSAID" has persisted for decades (see Sect. 2.1). As several NSAIDs are available without a prescription, patients take one of these supposedly harmless drugs (e.g., ibuprofen) for a long time without medical advice, thereby promoting development of serious ADRs (see Sects. 3.2 and 5.1). If, in contrast, the neutral term "cyclooxygenase inhibitors" is used to describe the mechanism of action of NSAIDs, these misunderstandings do not arise.

1.3   How Do Drugs Get to Market?

How Did Drug Development Work in the Past?

Summary

Development and approval of a drug is a long process. A distinction is made between a preclinical phase and three clinical phases. Only when a drug has cleared all of the hurdles does approval take place. After that, testing of the drug under real-world conditions begins. With newly approved drugs, there may be unforeseen ADRs or insufficient therapeutic efficacy that could lead to withdrawal of the drug. From the point of view of drug safety, patients are well advised if their doctor initially prescribes long-established drugs whose risks are well known. You should be cautious when buying drugs on the Internet or abroad.

Memo

- Tell your doctor or pharmacist about any ADRs.
- Take advantage of the advisory skills of your pharmacist.
- Never buy drugs from obscure sources.
- New drugs are not necessarily more effective than old drugs.
- New drugs are usually expensive.
- For many diseases, well-established drugs can be used.
- Particularly in the case of mental disorders, drugs must often be "tested".
- Do not read drug advertisements.
- Critically check the truthfulness of information about drugs on the Internet.
- An important current development is reuse of known drugs for new indications (repurposing).

Until the 1970s, drug development was not standardized. In many cases, drugs were tested on humans in various clinical situations on the basis of the results of animal experiments, or random observations were made on patients to whom certain drugs were administered. Self-trials or trials of drugs on family members (see Sect. 9.1) were common. This erratic process of drug development did, however, produce a number of valuable drugs, such as antipsychotics for treatment of schizophrenia (see Sect. 9.4), lithium for treatment of bipolar disorder (see Sect. 9.3), and methylphenidate for treatment of attention deficit–hyperactivity disorder (ADHD; see Sect. 9.1).

The Contergan® disaster at the end of the 1950s represented a turning point in drug development. Contergan®, containing thalidomide, was advertised as a "safe" drug for treatment of sleep disorders in pregnant women but caused severe malformations in embryos (e.g., phocomelia [severely shortened limbs]). These unanticipated effects were the reason for later, far-reaching changes in pharmaceutical law globally.

Caution When Buying Drugs Abroad

In several countries, you can buy certain drugs (e.g., analgesics [painkillers]) in unlimited quantities, or you can get highly effective drugs not only in pharmacies but also in drugstores or "health shops".

Be careful with supposedly "cheap" bulk purchases of drugs abroad. Many of the drugs on offer (e.g., painkillers) can cause serious ADRs if used in excess. Do not be misled by discounts ("buy one, get one free"). Discounts suggest that the drugs are harmless in double doses, but this is not the case. In some countries, the drugs offered are fakes. This applies, for example, to antibiotics (see Sect. 11.3) and, in particular, to drugs for erectile dysfunction (see Sect. 7.2). You must be aware of the possibility of counterfeits in the case of drugs that you obtain online from sources that are not clearly defined, other than reputable online pharmacies. If you obtain drugs from obscure sources, in the best case, you will lose your money and not have the desired effect. In the worst case, serious ADRs can result from toxic mixtures.

How Does Drug Development Work?

Figure 1.2 shows the process of modern drug development in the pharmaceutical industry. For such purposes, the companies have huge collections of pharmacologically active substances. Drug development is divided into a preclinical phase and three clinical phases. In the preclinical phase, the pharmacologically active substances are first investigated on cell components such as proteins and cultured cells. Computer methods play a role in drug

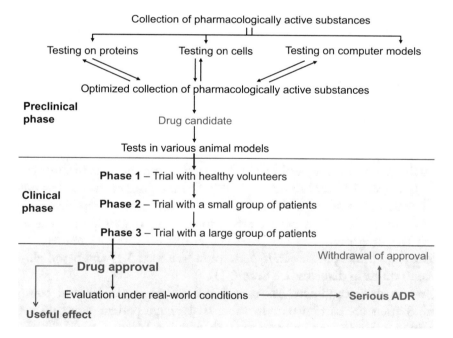

Fig. 1.2 Overview of drug development. A pharmacologically active substance becomes an approved drug in several steps. At each stage, the development can fail. In the case of serious adverse drug reactions (ADRs), the approval of a drug can be withdrawn. By observing beneficial effects and ADRs, everybody taking a drug can make a small contribution to drug safety and discovery of new indications (repurposing). Evaluation of randomly observed drug effects is an important source of improvements in drug therapy

development. At the end of this process, a small, optimized collection of drug candidates is developed for the specific target. In Sect. 1.4, these drug targets are discussed in detail.

In a further optimization process, a drug candidate is identified that not only has an appropriate therapeutic effect but also is likely to migrate easily through the body (Sect. 1.5). This candidate is then investigated in animal models for the respective disease. Every drug researcher (pharmacologist) knows that animal models have only limited informative value for a human disease, but well-designed animal experiments can be used to make a statement as to whether a certain drug could be effective in a human disease. As a rule, animal experiments are not carried out only in one animal species and only in one disease model. This increases the informative value of the studies. Well-designed experiments in mammals are an important part of drug development. They provide information on the dose of a drug candidate that can be safely tested in the clinical phase in human volunteers.

Drug researchers strive to obtain maximum information about the efficacy and safety of a drug before it is used in humans. This is in your best interests. Experiments in mammals are supplemented by studies in fish, worms, insects, and cultured cells. All of these studies add up to a complete picture.

You can be sure that animal testing is becoming more and more refined and improved, and that drug researchers are doing everything they can to reduce the number of animal tests and to establish replacement models (e.g., cultured artificial organs).

Once a drug candidate has cleared preclinical development, clinical testing begins. This takes place in three phases. In the first phase, the drug candidate is usually given to young healthy volunteers to determine its path through the body (see Sect. 1.5) and to detect ADRs. Once a drug candidate has passed this hurdle, it is tested for the first time in a small group of patients in the second phase. Here, it is particularly important to determine the extent to which the drug candidate has beneficial effects on certain parameters of a disease (e.g., blood pressure in hypertension [see Sect. 5.1] and blood glucose concentrations in diabetes [see Sect. 6.1]).

Once a drug candidate has passed this phase, expensive and complex phase 3 trials are carried out. In these trials, large patient populations are examined, often in many different locations (in multicenter trials). Here, the focus is no longer just on the analysis of laboratory values; it is also on "hard" end points in diseases, such as prolongation of life, improvement of quality of life, and prevention of secondary diseases. To assess the effect of the drug candidate, a proportion of the patients must be treated with a placebo (see Sect. 1.1). It is important that a known drug ("the gold standard") is investigated in parallel in another part of the patient population. From such comparisons, it can be concluded whether the new drug is superior to the old one. Often, however, this is not the case. The pharmaceutical industry then euphemistically speaks of the "noninferiority" of the new drug candidate. This results not in a better therapy for patients but in increasing costs in the health care system. The aim of clinical trials is to improve on an existing treatment option, not just to make a new drug that is equal to existing therapies.

A fundamental problem with phase 3 trials is that they are usually financed by the pharmaceutical industry, not by the public sector. Pharmaceutical companies have an interest in ensuring that a study turns out to be as positive as possible and that subsequent marketing of the drug is facilitated. Important points of criticism in many clinical studies are withholding (nonpublication) of unfavorable study results and lack of comparison between new drugs and the existing ones.

Lack of publication of negative trial results creates a bias in the scientific literature in favor of positive study results. This has been particularly evident in studies of drug therapy for depression (see Sect. 9.2).

If a drug candidate has successfully passed clinical phase 3, it becomes a "real" drug. The pharmaceutical manufacturer can apply for drug approval. Newly approved drugs almost always have a high price. Therefore, their prescribing should be weighed up carefully.

Real-World Testing of Drugs

Approval of a new drug marks the beginning of its real test. Clinical trials are conducted under well-controlled conditions with a lot of medical attention and often comfortable accommodation at hotel-like trial centers. In addition, the trials exclude many potential patients from the outset. However, such a selected group of trial subjects does not necessarily have much in common with the "real" patient population: real patients may forget to take their pills or accidentally take a double dose and take additional nonprescription drugs without medical consultation. Furthermore, they may have irregular lives, have concomitant diseases, and consume alcohol and tobacco. All of these factors can have profound effects on the efficacy of a drug but are not captured in clinical trials.

It is therefore not uncommon for a new drug with positive results in clinical trials to have a less convincing effect under real-world conditions or exhibit previously unobserved ADRs. In the worst case, a drug can be withdrawn from the market.

For example, after the market launch of the "new oral anticoagulants" (NOACs), which are factor Xa inhibitors (the prototype drug is rivaroxaban), these drugs were hailed as a breakthrough in treatment of myocardial infarction and strokes, and they were aggressively promoted. However, it has since become clear that the success of treatment depends greatly on patients taking the tablets regularly (see Sect. 5.2). If a patient accidentally forgets to take a tablet, the effect of the drug is quickly lost and a cardiovascular event may occur.

If your doctor prescribes you a newly approved drug, it is particularly important that you inform them of any ADR. By doing so, you can make an important contribution to drug safety. With newly approved drugs, we still have a lack of experience regarding efficacy and ADRs under "real-world conditions". Therefore, newly approved drugs should be used only with good justification. Evaluating a drug under "real-world conditions" is not easy, because there are many more variables than there are in clinical trials. Pharmaceutical companies try to address this by performing observational studies, but financial conflicts of interest involving the doctors participating in these observations often exist.

Off-Label Use of Drugs

Drugs are approved for the indications investigated in the clinical trials. However, your doctor may prescribe a drug for another indication. Of course, they must inform you accordingly. Off-label use of drugs (i.e., their use beyond the scope of the marketing authorization) represents both an opportunity and a risk. Particularly in the case of mental disorders (and especially in child and adolescent psychiatry), it is common to "test" drugs. Over the years, the strategy of off-label use has led to a situation in which the areas of application of "antidepressants", "antiepileptics", and "antipsychotics" have expanded and mixed to such an extent that the traditional drug class designations are no longer appropriate (see Sect. 1.2 and Chaps. 8 and 9).

Drug Repurposing

The advantage of drugs that have been approved for many years is that their efficacy, ADRs, and interactions are well known. This increases drug safety. These drugs have overcome all of the hurdles of drug approval and passed tests under real-world conditions over many years.

This broad knowledge of a drug can be used to apply it in completely different diseases. This is known as repurposing. Such repurposing can follow from theoretical considerations, and sometimes chance helps. For example, it was found by chance that in patients with type 2 diabetes, the antidiabetic drug metformin improved not only the symptoms of diabetes but also the symptoms of polycystic ovary syndrome, which was present in some patients at the same time. Currently, drug repurposing is playing a major role in treatment of the viral disease COVID-19 (see Sect. 11.3).

If you notice an unexpected positive effect of a drug on you, inform your doctor or pharmacist. Perhaps you hold the key to a new therapy in your hands that will benefit many patients.

Getting Information on Drugs

The information content of drug advertising is usually low. In professional journals for doctors and pharmacists, the positive aspects of the drug are emphasized in large print with suggestive statements and, above all, photos. In contrast, information on ADRs and costs is shown in such small print at the bottom of the advertisement that the text is hardly readable.

The situation is similar with drug advertising targeted at patients. Often, unrealistic promises are made about positive effects that cannot be kept. The fact that patients lack specialized knowledge is consciously used for profit maximization. One often looks in vain for scientific proof of the effectiveness of drugs in advertising targeted at patients.

Anyone who wants to obtain serious information about drugs must read textbooks written by recognized experts. For further information, it is essential to read scientific reviews and original research papers that have been conscientiously examined by experts.

Nowadays, many patients use the Internet to obtain information on health topics and drugs. The problem with such information sources is that the authors of the texts are often not personally identifiable. This makes it difficult to identify conflicts of interest (e.g., sales interests for a particular brand-name drug) and to assess the authors' qualifications. The current trend in medicine can be seen on the Internet: everything is becoming much more specialized and detailed, but the context is getting lost. Therefore, the primary aim of this book is to show you relations between different medical specialties. Please pay attention to the cross-references between the individual sections.

Be critical of information from the Internet. Ask who the author is and whether there may be conflicts of interest. A fancy website is no guarantee of serious content. In this author's experience, information on drugs in the online encyclopedia Wikipedia is reliable. It contains many references for further reading. However, pharmacological terms are not used consistently, and relations between topics are presented only in a limited way. For patients, the information available in Wikipedia is often difficult to understand and too extensive.

1.4 How Do Drugs Work in Your Body?

Summary

Drugs change the function of the body's cells. In many diseases, the aim is to restore a disturbed balance of bodily functions through drug therapy. This can easily be imagined with the help of a scale, as you will find in many figures in this book. Important drug targets are (1) receptors, (2) enzymes, (3) pumps, (4) channels, and (5) the cell nucleus. Some drugs have many targets. This can be advantageous or disadvantageous, depending on the disease. In many cases, ADRs can be derived from the mechanism of action.

Memo

- In many diseases, the balance of body functions is disturbed.
- Drugs are used to restore the balance.
- Receptors, enzymes, pumps, channels, and the cell nucleus are important drug targets.
- Receptors are activated by agonists; antagonists prevent activation of receptors.
- "Good" examples of drugs with only one target are the setrons, used to treat migraine attacks.
- "Bad" examples of drugs with only one target are the antihistamines, used to treat allergic shock.
- "Good" examples of drugs with numerous targets are the antipsychotics, used to treat schizophrenia.
- "Bad" examples of drugs with numerous targets are the nonselective beta blockers, previously used to treat cardiovascular disease.
- In many cases, ADRs are explained by the mechanism of action of a drug.

What Is the Basis of Drug Effects?

Our body consists of organ systems (e.g., the cardiovascular system, central nervous system, and digestive system). Each organ is composed of cell assemblies (tissues) consisting of cells of a certain type (e.g., nerve cells and muscle cells). Drugs influence the function of cells by binding to specific targets. The drug and its target must fit like a lock and its key.

In diseases, cell functions are out of balance. The aim of drug therapy is to restore the body's balance (homeostasis) as far as possible. The disturbed balance in diseases is shown in the form of a scale in several figures in this book (see Figs. 3.2, 3.3, 6.3, 8.1, 8.2, 10.1, and 11.3).

Drug therapy influences cell functions. Every cell has the same basic structure. Figure 1.3 shows a cell and how it is influenced by drugs. Each cell is surrounded by a membrane that separates it from the outside. Cells carry

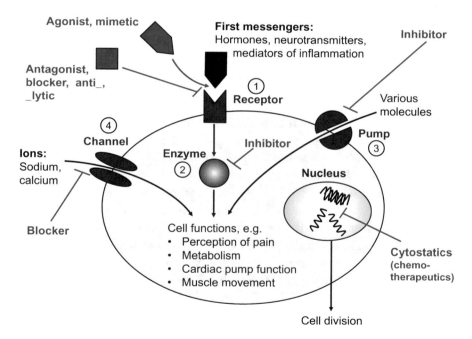

Fig. 1.3 Overview of the cell structure and drug targets. Important drug targets are marked by the *circled numbers 1–5*. For some drug classes with a clearly defined mechanism (e.g., receptor antagonists), quite different terms are used for historical reasons, which at first sight have nothing to do with each other. This can lead to confusion. To ensure the broadest possible comprehensibility, traditional terms are used in this book, despite all of the associated problems. The tables and the glossary (see the Appendix) mention the mechanistic terms

receptors (target no. 1), which are activated by "first messengers" (hormones, neurotransmitters, and mediators of inflammation) and transmit signals into the cell. First messengers are agonists that bind to receptors and activate them. Activated receptors generate "second messengers" that regulate enzymes (target no. 2), which control our metabolism.

Cells have pumps (target no. 3) that transport nutrients and neurotransmitters into the cells. Furthermore, nerve cells and muscle cells have channels (target no. 4) in the membrane. Influx of sodium and calcium excites these cells. Finally, cells have a nucleus (target no. 5) to duplicate our genetic material (deoxyribonucleic acid [DNA]) and to initiate cell division (cell reproduction). Depending on the specialization of a cell, it performs different functions: nerve cells mediate perception of pain, liver cells secure energy supply in the body, and heart muscle cells pump blood.

Receptors as Target No. 1

In Fig. 1.3, a receptor is marked as target no. 1 for drugs. Over 1000 different receptors are present in our body, and they are activated by different first messengers. Receptors are important targets for drugs. We distinguish between two classes of drugs that target receptors:

(a) **Agonists:** They activate receptors in the same way as the body's own first messengers. Traditionally, receptor agonists are called "_mimetics" (e.g., beta sympathomimetics; see Sects. 4.1 and 4.2).

(b) **Antagonists:** They bind to receptors without activating them. Antagonists compete with agonists for binding to receptors; they thereby prevent activation of receptors by the body's own messenger substances (agonists) and inhibit cell functions. The term "blocker" is commonly used for antagonists (e.g., angiotensin receptor blockers and beta blockers; see Sect. 5.1), as are the word stems "anti_" (e.g., antihistamines [see Sect. 4.1] and antipsychotics [see Sect. 9.4]) and "_lytic" (e.g., parasympatholytics; see Sects. 3.1, 3.3, 4.1, 4.2, 8.1, 9.2, 9.4, and 10.1). Thus, differently spelled terms describe a common mechanism of action.

For better comprehensibility, traditional drug class designations for agonists and antagonists are used in this book. In the glossary, the more recent terms are mentioned.

Enzymes as Target No. 2

In Fig. 1.3, an enzyme is marked as target no. 2 for drugs. In the human body, there are almost 3000 enzymes, which are responsible for all metabolic processes. Numerous drugs inhibit enzymes. These drugs are called inhibitors. The most familiar examples are the NSAIDs. They inhibit an enzyme called cyclooxygenase (COX) and thus inhibit formation of prostaglandins in the body. Reduced prostaglandin synthesis results in relief from pain, inflammation, and fever (see Sect. 2.1). Therefore, NSAIDs are commonly used. However, if taken for a long time, NSAIDs can cause high blood pressure and peptic ulcer disease (PUD; see Sect. 3.2).

The effects of certain cytostatics (chemotherapeutic agents, which inhibit cell division), antibiotics, and antiviral drugs are based on enzyme inhibition. Enzymes that play a role in cell growth and division are targeted in the fight against cancer (see Sect. 11.1). Inhibition of bacterial or viral enzymes is used to treat corresponding infections (see Sect. 11.3).

Pumps as Target No. 3

In Fig. 1.3, a pump is marked as target no. 3 for drugs. We have hundreds of different pumps in our body. They are responsible for transporting nutrients, neurotransmitters, and drugs. Several important drugs inhibit pumps—for example, pumps that reabsorb the neurotransmitters serotonin and norepinephrine into nerve cells. The corresponding pump inhibitors increase the amounts of serotonin and norepinephrine available outside nerve cells. This is an important approach in drug therapy for depression, anxiety, and obsessive–compulsive disorders, which are characterized by deficiencies in these neurotransmitters (see Sect. 9.2). Many cancer cells have pumps that eliminate cytostatics from cells. This makes the cancer cells insensitive to the drug, and the cancer continues to grow again. This is a major problem in cancer therapy (see Sect. 11.1).

Channels as Target No. 4

In Fig. 1.3, a channel is marked as drug target no. 4. There are hundreds of different channels in the human body. They mediate influx of ions into cells. Sodium and calcium channels are the most important channels for drug therapy. These channels mediate excitation of nerve and muscle cells. Calcium channel blockers are used in treatment of high blood pressure and many neurological and mental disorders (see Sect. 5.1 and Chaps. 8 and 9). Sodium channel blockers play a major role in treatment of neurological and mental disorders (see Chaps. 8 and 9).

The Cell Nucleus as Target No. 5

In Fig. 1.3, the cell nucleus is marked as target no. 5 for drugs. In the cell nucleus, DNA is replicated and thus cell division is initiated. In the human body, cell division is particularly important for blood cells, immune cells, and epithelial cells (which are present in hair, skin, and mucous membranes). If cell division proceeds in an uncontrolled manner, a malignant tumor (cancer) develops. Therefore, drugs that inhibit cell division (cytostatics) are the backbone of cancer therapy (see Sect. 11.1). These drugs target the cell nucleus. However, cytostatics also inhibit proliferation of normal cells, causing hair loss, digestive disorders, and immune deficiency. In low doses, certain cytostatics are used to treat autoimmune diseases (see Sect. 11.2).

Is It Good or Bad if a Drug Has Only One Target?

The decisive factor is the specific situation in the respective disease. Let's have a look at the following examples.

Triptans are serotonin-1 receptor agonists and prevent release of a mediator of inflammation in arteries beneath the skull. Triptans do not affect other targets. In this case, it is "good" that the drug affects only one receptor, because it has a convincing therapeutic effect in an acute migraine attack (see Sect. 2.1) with only a few ADRs.

On the other hand, it can be "bad" if a drug has only one target. Let's look at the antihistamines used in the treatment of allergic shock. In the past, this treatment was commonplace. However, in allergic shock, mediators of inflammation other than histamine play roles as well (see Sect. 4.1). Therefore, giving a patient only antihistamines during a severe allergic reaction provides little relief, since the effects of the other mediators of inflammation are not inhibited. Therefore, allergic shock is treated with epinephrine (adrenaline). It abrogates the effects of histamine and other mediators of inflammation, and it is highly effective.

Is It Good or Bad if a Drug Has Many Targets?

Again, it depends on the disease. In schizophrenia, for example, the function of various neurotransmitter receptors is exaggerated. Consequently, drugs that are antagonists at many neurotransmitter receptors have good antipsychotic effects (see Sect. 9.4). This is an important example of how it can be good if a drug has many targets.

And here an example of how it can be "bad": In the past, cardiovascular diseases used to be treated with the "nonselective beta blocker" propranolol. It blocks all beta receptors. However, for treatment of cardiovascular diseases, only the beta-1 receptor must be blocked (antagonized). Blocking the beta-2 receptor causes numerous ADRs, such as a risk of asthma attacks, cold fingers, and undetected hypoglycemia (low blood sugar) in patients with diabetes. Because of this bad situation, "selective beta-1 blockers" were developed, which in therapeutic doses no longer have the unpleasant effects of nonselective beta blockers.

How Do Adverse Drug Reactions Occur?

In many cases, an ADR can be derived from the mechanism of action, as the following examples show.

Methylphenidate is used to treat ADHD (see Sect. 9.1). Known ADRs include an increase in blood pressure and loss of appetite. In addition, the beneficial effect of methylphenidate decreases significantly when it is taken in high doses and without a break. How do these ADRs, which seem so different, come about? Methylphenidate enhances release of neurotransmitters that increase attention (desired). Unfortunately, it also increases blood pressure and inhibits appetite (both undesired). When the neurotransmitter stores are depleted (like a flat smartphone battery), they must first be slowly restored before they work properly again. This is the reason why medication breaks ("drug holidays") are necessary during methylphenidate therapy.

Antidepressants from the class of selective serotonin reuptake inhibitors (SSRIs) increase the amount of serotonin in the brain and improve depressed mood (see Sect. 9.2). But serotonin plays a role in regulation of the cardiovascular and gastrointestinal systems. Too much serotonin in these systems leads to high blood pressure or nausea and vomiting as ADRs.

It is therefore worthwhile to understand how a drug works, as this mechanism provides a good explanation for many ADRs. Knowledge of the causes of ADRs will help you to accept the disadvantages of a necessary treatment, to reduce your fears, and to optimize the therapy together with your doctor (e.g., by adjusting the dose).

In many cases, it will be impossible to provide perfect drug therapy. It will often be a matter of finding a compromise between desired effects and ADRs. So, be realistic with your expectations of drug therapy. This is especially true if you are receiving treatment for a mental disorder. Observe your body because, as your condition changes, the therapeutic effects of the drug and the associated ADRs may change as well.

The optimal drug therapy for you may need to be adjusted regularly. The extent of the ADRs that you must put up with depends on the severity of the disease. This can best be explained using cancer as an example. Cancer is a matter of life or death. Cytostatics (which act on target no. 5 in Fig. 1.3) do not distinguish between healthy cells and cancer cells. They destroy both types of cells (see Sect. 11.1). Therefore, cytostatics cause many ADRs. For treatment of a mild condition such as a tension headache, however, the drug that is used must not trigger severe ADRs (see Sect. 2.1).

Unfortunately, the occurrence of ADRs is too rarely explained to the patient in routine medical practice. Often doctors supposedly do not have enough time, although it would be time well spent and would increase the patient's adherence to therapy. Package leaflets merely list ADRs in a catalogue-like manner without explaining how they occur. If you know why each effect occurs, it will be easier for you to take a drug with significant ADRs regularly.

1.5   How Do Drugs Travel Through the Body?

Summary

Drugs make a long journey through the body; whenever possible, they are given by mouth. Drug absorption occurs in the small intestine and is dependent on food intake. After absorption in the small intestine, drugs are distributed into the organs and cause therapeutic effects and ADRs by binding to their targets. Drugs used in the treatment of neurological and mental disorders must be fat soluble to reach the brain. Most drugs are broken down in the liver. This can lead to interactions between different drugs and food components. Most drugs are excreted by the kidneys. In the case of impaired kidney function, the doses of many drugs must be reduced.

Memo

- Pay close attention to whether a drug must be taken on an empty stomach or with food.
- In the case of a drug with many ADRs, the drug concentration is measured in the blood.
- To avoid interactions, you should take as few drugs as possible. This includes drugs that you buy over the counter.
- Herbal drugs can cause serious interactions.
- Special dietary habits can influence the effects of drugs.
- In infants and young children, caution is needed because drugs can enter the immature brain.
- The risk of ADRs is high in patients with chronic kidney failure.
- The fewer drugs you take, the lower the risks of ADRs and drug interactions.
- Drugs with different areas of application can interact with each other.

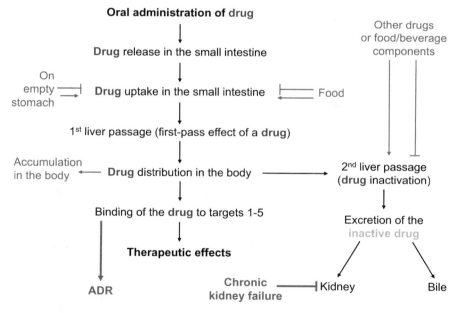

Fig. 1.4 The path of a drug through the body. Shown in *green* are factors that can interfere with the path of a drug through the body. Some of these examples are explained in section "The Path of a Drug Through the Body". In patients with chronic kidney failure, the doses of many drugs must be reduced. The term "ADR" (adverse drug reaction) is explained in Fig. 1.1, Fig. 1.2, and Table 2.2. The term "target" is explained in Fig. 1.3

The Path of a Drug Through the Body

Figure 1.4 shows the path of a drug through the body. Most drugs are taken by mouth (orally). In infants and children, sweetened juices are often used (e.g., paracetamol [acetaminophen] juice for treatment of fever; see Sect. 2.1) to mask the bitter taste of many drugs. For elderly people with difficulties in swallowing, drops are suitable (e.g., metamizole or tramadol drops to treat pain; see Sects. 2.1 and 2.2). After passing through the esophagus and stomach, most drugs are absorbed into the body via the small intestine.

Drugs for treatment of neurological and mental disorders must reach the brain by crossing the blood–brain barrier. For this purpose, the drug must be fat soluble, small, and uncharged. An example of a pharmacologically active substance with such properties, which everyone knows of, is ethanol in alcoholic beverages.

The duration of the effect of a drug depends on its half-life. The half-life defines the time in which half of the amount of an absorbed drug is degraded or excreted. The half-lives of different drugs differ enormously; they range from a few minutes (e.g., the half-life of glycerol trinitrate) to several years (e.g., the half-lives of bisphosphonates; see Sect. 6.3). For emergency situations, drugs with a short duration of action are preferred; for long-term therapy, those with a long duration of action are preferred. The aim is to prevent a drug from accumulating in the body and thus causing problems over a long period. A good example of a problematic drug is amiodarone, which can be used for tachycardia (atrial fibrillation and ventricular tachycardia; see Sect. 5.2). Amiodarone takes months to be excreted from the body, and so it is possible to experience ADRs long after treatment has ended.

After distribution in the body, a drug binds to its targets and causes therapeutic effects and ADRs (see Sect. 1.4). The drug then enters the liver again and is broken down (inactivated) by enzymes in various steps. If the liver breaks down only one drug, usually no problems are observed. But as soon as you take several drugs, there may be competition for their breakdown, which, therefore, proceeds more slowly. As a result, you will notice prolongation of the effects of the different drugs and/or increases in the ADRs associated with them. The biggest mistake you or your doctor can make in such a situation is trying to treat this type of ADR with another drug, because then your body will get even more out of balance.

Some drugs inhibit breakdown of other drugs, thereby increasing those other drug's effects. Conversely, some drugs activate the liver and thus accelerate breakdown of other drugs, reducing those other drugs' effects. So, it can become complicated when even just two drugs are taken.

After drugs have been broken down in the liver, they are excreted in the bile and above all in the kidneys. With age, the function of the kidney and hence its ability to excrete drugs decrease. Inadequately treated high blood pressure (see Sect. 5.1) and diabetes in particular (see Sect. 6.1) impair kidney function.

With decreasing kidney function, drugs remain longer in the body and are more likely to cause ADRs, especially when several drugs are given. In elderly people, who often take several drugs, it is important to consider which drug can be discontinued to avoid problems. The basic rule is "less is more!" To adjust the dose, the kidney function of older patients is measured (by measuring the creatinine level in the blood or, more precisely, the creatinine excretion from the body over 24 hours). For this measurement, urine output over a 24-hour period must be collected and analyzed.

Other Forms of Drug Administration

In some cases (e.g., use of glycerol trinitrate in angina pectoris, scopolamine in motion sickness, or estrogen in hormone replacement therapy [see Sect. 7.1]), a drug is degraded during its first liver passage after oral administration. This is referred to as a first-pass effect of a drug. In such cases, alternative routes of administration (e.g., an oral spray or a skin patch with a drug depot) are used.

Some drugs—such as epinephrine (adrenaline; see Sect. 4.1), insulin (see Sect. 6.1), certain antibiotics (see Sect. 11.3), and drugs used to treat cancer and autoimmune diseases (see Sects. 11.1 and 11.2)—are water soluble or sensitive to gastric acid, so they cannot be absorbed into the body when given orally. They are therefore administered by bypassing the intestine (parenteral administration). Drugs can be administered into a vein (intravenously [IV]), under the skin (subcutaneously [SC]), or into a muscle (intramuscularly [IM]). The onset of action is quickest with intravenous administration, as the blood circulation distributes the drug throughout the body within a few seconds. This is used, for example, in emergency treatment of allergic shock (see Sect. 4.1). In some cases (e.g., pain therapy with fentanyl), a rapid onset of action can be achieved by administering the drug into the nose (intranasally [IN]) or by dissolving drug-containing lozenges under the tongue or in the cheek (lingually and buccally).

Therapeutic Drug Monitoring

Some diseases require use of drugs that are effective but have serious ADRs. The aim of drug therapy is to achieve the best possible therapeutic effect without ADRs becoming too severe (see Sect. 1.4). Over time, experience has been gained as to the blood levels of drugs at which the best therapeutic effects are achieved. Blood is taken from the patient, and the concentration (level) of the drug is determined in the blood. This is referred to as therapeutic drug monitoring (TDM). If the drug level is too low or too high, the dose must be increased or decreased, respectively. Thus, your doctor has a good tool to increase drug safety. TDM can be used to check whether you are taking your drugs regularly. If the levels are unrealistically low, this is an indication of a lack of adherence to therapy. You should tell your doctor honestly why you are not taking your drug. In many cases, it is possible to find an alternative for you.

TDM is particularly common in epilepsy (see Sect. 8.1), bipolar disorder (see Sect. 9.3), schizophrenia (see Sect. 9.4), autoimmune disorders (see Sect. 11.2), organ transplantation (see Sect. 11.2), and some serious infectious diseases (see Sect. 11.3).

In the case of the vitamin K antagonist warfarin, which is used for prevention of strokes and myocardial infarction, indirect TDM is used. The effect of the drug is determined by the clotting ability of the blood (which is measured as the international normalized ratio [INR] value; see Sect. 5.2). Indirect TDM is performed in diabetes by assessing the effect of the drug on the blood glucose concentration (see Sect. 6.1). In the case of respiratory disease, the effect of the drug is measured indirectly by lung function parameters (e.g., peak flow; see Sects. 4.1 and 4.2). In all cases, the patient can actively participate in indirect TDM. This strengthens personal responsibility and increases adherence to therapy.

Risks of Taking Many Drugs (Polypharmacy)

In certain situations, it makes sense to take several drugs. Examples are treatment of high blood pressure (see Sect. 5.1), prevention of heart attacks and strokes (see Sect. 5.2), cancer treatment (see Sect. 11.1), and the treatment of autoimmune diseases (see Sect. 11.2).

Problems often arise if a patient has several diseases and is prescribed drugs from different specialists without the latter having an overview of the patient's entire medication. Therefore, it is important that you carry an up-to-date list of all of your drugs. This includes those you have purchased without a doctor's prescription. Comprehensive databases where your doctor or pharmacist can look up drug interactions are available. Your responsibility is to keep your doctor and pharmacist informed about your medication. Three examples are provided below to make you aware of the issues.

Example 1: Dangerous Herbal Drugs

Let us assume that you take the immunosuppressive drug ciclosporin (see Sect. 11.2) because of psoriasis, an autoimmune disease. The disease is putting a lot of strain on you (your skin itches, flakes, and is red), and not everything is going well in your private and professional life. You feel depressed but do not want to see a psychiatrist. You have read on the Internet that St. John's wort extracts are supposedly effective against depression, and you therefore buy St. John's wort capsules from an online mail order company. In your opinion, such herbal drugs are much better than "chemicals" anyway. You then take the St. John's wort capsules for 3 weeks and are disappointed to find that your depression has not improved. Moreover, your psoriasis has worsened considerably. What happened? St. John's wort extracts contain a pharmacologically active substance (hyperforin), which activates the liver and causes ciclosporin to be broken down and removed from the body more quickly. Therefore, your psoriasis has worsened. In addition, there is a lack of convincing evidence that St. John's wort extracts are effective in treating depression. You should therefore discuss your depressive mood with your doctor. He will prescribe an effective antidepressant that does not interact with ciclosporin (see Sect. 9.2).

Example 2: The Risks of Consulting Many Doctors

You had a stroke 3 years ago and have since been treated by your neurologist with warfarin, a vitamin K antagonist (see Sect. 5.2). The doctor checks your INR regularly and everything is fine. Suddenly, during the flu season, you develop a fever and a cough with purulent sputum. You suspect that you have contracted bronchitis. You make an appointment with a lung specialist. He listens to your lungs, takes an X-ray, and confirms the suspected diagnosis of bronchitis. As you are going on vacation, you push the doctor to prescribe you an antibiotic. You do not mention that you are taking warfarin, because you assume that this belongs in a "different box". The lung specialist prescribes the antibiotic clarithromycin for 5 days, which is suitable for bronchitis. You tolerate the antibiotic well, but suddenly, on the fourth day of treatment, you get such a severe nosebleed that you are taken to the emergency room. You must be hospitalized and will now miss your vacation. What happened? Clarithromycin inhibits breakdown of warfarin in the liver. The increase in the warfarin level in the body has reduced the blood's ability to clot to such an extent that spontaneous nosebleeds have occurred. You've been lucky in this case. A life-threatening bleeding event could have occurred. The whole episode would not have happened if you had told the lung specialist that you were taking warfarin. Then he would have picked out an antibiotic (such as amoxicillin) that does not interact with the breakdown of warfarin. This example highlights your responsibility as a patient to fully inform the doctors you consult about all of the drugs you are taking.

Example 3: Long-Term Therapy with Ibuprofen
You have been treated for a year with an ACE inhibitor (ramipril) and a diuretic (furosemide) for moderate heart failure (see Sect. 5.3). With this therapy, you can manage all daily activities. Your doctor has told you to exercise your heart as much as possible and to go for regular walks. In spring, your right knee starts to ache while you are walking. You know that you have signs of wear and tear (osteoarthritis). You read in a newspaper advertisement that ibuprofen is supposed to be good for such joint complaints, and that 400-mg tablets are available over the counter (see Sect. 2.1). You get the ibuprofen and do not ask what the correct dose is. You do not consult your doctor, because you assume that an over-the-counter drug is harmless. You notice that taking a 400-mg ibuprofen tablet three times per day helps you a little, but if you instead take a 600-mg dose (one whole 400-mg tablet plus another half tablet, divided at the fracture groove) three times per day, your knee is much better, and you can walk for longer distances. Everything seems fine, and you feel as though you're doing something good for your knee and your heart with ibuprofen. However, as the summer progresses, you become increasingly sleepy, your physical performance deteriorates, and you need to go to the toilet less often. Soon, you are so weak that you can no longer stand up, and your daughter must call an ambulance. At the hospital, you are diagnosed with acute kidney failure. What happened? Continuous ibuprofen treatment of patients with cardiovascular disease is dangerous (see Sects. 2.1, 5.1, and 5.3). Ibuprofen has reduced blood flow to your kidneys to such an extent that they have stopped functioning. The risk of kidney failure from ibuprofen and other NSAIDs is particularly high when ACE inhibitors and diuretics are given at the same time. This example shows how dangerous it is to take over-the-counter (and thus supposedly harmless) painkillers on a long-term basis. If ibuprofen is stopped, kidney failure can usually be reversed. If you had talked to your doctor or pharmacist about your joint pain, they could have found another painkiller for you (e.g., paracetamol [acetaminophen] or metamizole [dipyrone]) that is not harmful to the kidneys (see Sect. 2.1).

Interaction of Foods with Drugs

Numerous foods interact with drugs. One example is ethanol in alcoholic beverages. You all know from experience that after a glass of champagne or wine on an empty stomach, you will feel a pronounced effect of the ethanol within 5–10 minutes. On the other hand, if you drink the alcohol as part of a solid meal, it takes much longer for the ethanol to start working, and the maximum effect is much weaker. But the effect lasts longer. This example shows that food intake can delay the absorption of drugs. For many diseases that are treated with long-term medication, this is usually not a problem.

However, thyroid hormones for hypothyroidism (see Sect. 6.2), bisphosphonates for osteoporosis (see Sect. 6.3), and proton pump inhibitors (PPIs) for gastroesophageal reflux disease (GERD; see Sect. 3.1) must be taken on an empty stomach to ensure therapeutic effects without ADRs.

Use of calcium supplements to prevent osteoporosis is popular (see Sect. 6.3). However, calcium inhibits absorption of certain antibiotics (tetracyclines and fluoroquinolones; see Sect. 11.3) into the body because calcium forms insoluble precipitates with these drugs. Similar problems arise when calcium-containing foods such as milk and dairy products (e.g., yoghurt and cheese) are combined with certain antibiotics. It is therefore essential to check for any incompatibilities between calcium and each drug you are taking. The practical solution to the problem is simple. You must keep a gap of at least 2 hours between the intake of the drug and that of calcium. Then both will be absorbed into the body.

Other problems in the interaction between diet and certain drugs may arise if you follow a particular diet or if you have any preferences and therefore consume large amounts of a particular food. The following examples illustrate these points.

Example 1: Too Much Grapefruit Juice May Affect Your Heart
Grapefruit juice contains the bitter substance naringin, which inhibits breakdown of various drugs in the liver. As a result, the effects of these drugs last longer or the higher drug concentrations in the body cause ADRs. For example, life-threatening forms of tachycardia can occur with heavy consumption of grapefruit juice and concomitant treatment with certain antidepressants, antipsychotics (see Sects. 9.2 and 9.4), or antibiotics (see Sect. 11.3).

Example 2: Superfoods Can Cause Bleeding
Goji berries are mythicized as a superfood. The term "superfood" suggests health- and performance-promoting effects on the body and thus motivates you to consume large quantities of the food. If you eat large quantities of goji berries, various active substances contained in them can, for example, inhibit breakdown of the anticoagulant warfarin and thus cause severe bleeding (see "Example 2: The Risks of Consulting Many Doctors" above). So, eat goji berries sparingly.

> **Example 3: A Deadly Vegan Diet**
> Kale, white cabbage, and broccoli enjoy reputations as healthy foods. Their high popularity is due to the fact they contain large amounts of vitamin K. This vitamin is important for formation of certain blood-clotting factors, aids in hemostasis, and thus contributes to the body's natural protection against excessive bleeding from injury. However, if a patient is treated with the anticoagulant warfarin, which is a vitamin K antagonist (see Sect. 5.2), the "good" vitamin K competes with the drug and leads to increased formation of clotting factors. The result can be a heart attack or a stroke. Hence, vitamin K can become a killer (see "Example 2: The Risks of Consulting Many Doctors" above).

These few examples show that excessive consumption of supposedly healthy foods can cause considerable problems in combination with certain drugs. It is therefore important to check for each drug's incompatibilities and interactions with food. You can reduce the risk of unexpected interactions between foods and drugs by avoiding an unbalanced diet.

Reduce Drug Doses in Kidney Failure

The kidney is responsible for excretion of many drugs. Accordingly, if your kidney is damaged, your doctor must reduce the doses of such drugs. In addition, the number of different drugs that are administered should be reduced to a minimum so they do not compete for excretion in the weakened kidney. Drugs whose doses need to be reduced include the antiviral drug aciclovir for herpes zoster (shingles; see Sect. 11.3), metformin for type 2 diabetes (see Sect. 6.1), lithium for bipolar disorder (see Sect. 9.3), and methotrexate (MTX) for autoimmune diseases (see Sect. 11.2).

If you have impaired kidney function and are taking one of these drugs, you should inform each of your doctors to prevent ADRs when you are being prescribed another drug. Aciclovir is prescribed by dermatologists and neurologists, metformin by internists, lithium by psychiatrists, and methotrexate by rheumatologists. Often doctors are not aware of the risks that can arise when they prescribe one of these drugs if another doctor prescribes another drug that is excreted through the kidneys. Numerous avoidable deaths from accidental overdoses or additional use of other renally excreted drugs (particularly methotrexate [see Sect. 11.2]) have occurred.

The most important contribution you can make to drug safety in the case of impaired kidney function is to refrain from taking NSAIDs such as ibuprofen. "Example 3: Long-Term Therapy with Ibuprofen" (above) shows how dangerous long-term use of these drugs can be (see Sect. 2.1). NSAIDs should not be prescribed to patients with impaired kidney function. For pain and inflammation, other drugs that are not harmful to the kidneys are available (see Sects. 2.1, 2.2, and 11.2).

Treating Infants and Young Children

Infants and young children are not small adults. For infants and young children, you cannot simply use a percentage dose that corresponds to the body weight of an adult. In many cases, the doses of drugs used for children in relation to their body weight are higher than those used for adults (for a prime example, describing fever reduction with paracetamol [acetaminophen] suppositories, see Sect. 2.1). Certain drugs (especially benzodiazepines and non-benzodiazepines [Z-drugs]) with a sedative effect in adults can cause agitation in infants and young children, and they should therefore be avoided (see Sect. 8.2).

Normally, the blood–brain barrier is effective in preventing passage into the brain of drugs that are supposed to exert an effect only outside the brain. However, the blood–brain barrier of infants and young children is immature. In infants and young children, decongestant nasal drops (the prototype drug is xylometazoline) or drugs that relieve vomiting (the prototype drug is metoclopramide; see Sects. 3.1 and 3.3) can enter the brain more easily than they can in schoolchildren, adolescents, and adults; thus, they can cause severe ADRs.

Decongestant nose drops can cause high blood pressure. Therefore, the basic rule is that decongestant nasal drops for adults should never be given to infants or young children. Special decongestant nasal drops for babies and young children, with a lower drug dose than that used in adults, are available.

Metoclopramide can cause facial twitching and grimacing (similar to Tourette syndrome). While these symptoms are usually harmless and transient, they are socially disruptive. Facial twitching after consumption of metoclopramide is a common reason for parents to take their children to the emergency room. Because of its ADRs, metoclopramide should not be used in infants or children. Treatment of nausea and vomiting (often coupled with diarrhea; see Sect. 3.3) focuses on administration of electrolyte solutions (available in different flavors for children) and slow reintroduction of normal food.

2

Painkillers (Analgesics)

Abstract Pain is an unpleasant sensation with a high therapeutic priority. This chapter gives an overview of how pain is generated and processed in the body and what treatment options we have. Many more options for treating pain than the classic opioid and nonopioid analgesics are available. For most types of pain, a good treatment can be found, depending on the cause and severity. One focus of the chapter is a comparison of the three main nonopioid analgesics: ibuprofen, paracetamol (acetaminophen), and metamizole (dipyrone). Each of these three drugs has advantages and disadvantages. Opioid analgesics are often prescribed for more severe pain. We distinguish between analgesics with low efficacy (tramadol), medium efficacy (buprenorphine), and high efficacy (fentanyl and morphine). Opioid analgesics cause constipation, which must be treated. In high doses, opioid analgesics can cause respiratory failure. Contrary to widespread opinion, opioid analgesics do not pose a major risk of addiction when used properly.

2.1 Overview and Nonopioid Analgesics

Summary

Pain is an unpleasant sensation. Pain is transmitted from its origin in the body by peripheral nerves to the spinal cord and from there to the brain. Depending on the type and cause of the pain, different drugs are used for treatment. After an introduction to pain treatment principles, this section focuses on the commonly used nonopioid analgesics ibuprofen, paracetamol (acetaminophen), and metamizole (dipyrone). These three drugs have different pharmacological profiles and are associated with different adverse drug reactions (ADRs).

> **Memo**
>
> - Pain is treated with different drug classes, depending on the cause.
> - Analgesics are divided into nonopioid analgesics and opioid analgesics.
> - The main nonopioid analgesics are ibuprofen, paracetamol (acetaminophen), and metamizole (dipyrone).
> - Ibuprofen has analgesic, anti-inflammatory, and antipyretic effects. It can cause peptic ulcer disease (PUD) and increase blood pressure.
> - Paracetamol (acetaminophen) has analgesic and antipyretic effects. It can cause liver damage if overdosed.
> - Metamizole (dipyrone) relieves pain, especially colic pain, and reduces fever. It can (rarely) cause white blood cell depletion and allergic shock.
> - Coxibs are not a good alternative to ibuprofen, because they increase the risks of heart attacks and strokes.

2.2   How Pain Arises and How It Is Assessed

Pain is an unpleasant sensation with many causes. Depending on the cause and type, different drug classes are used to treat pain. Figure 2.1 shows an overview of the origin and transmission of pain, as well as the various targets of different drug classes.

In most cases, pain is caused by tissue damage. Cramps of internal organs (colics), vasodilation (migraine), and bone metastases in cancer can cause pain as well. Pain receptors are excited and send a signal through pain-conducting nerve cells to the spinal cord and ultimately to the brain. Damage to or malfunctioning of nerve cells can trigger pain. This is called neuropathy.

Perception and subjective assessment of pain take place in the brain. Since pain cannot be measured objectively and each patient has an individual assessment of pain, it is helpful to use a pain scale with numerical values ranging from 0 (no pain) to 10 (the strongest pain imaginable).

Different Painkillers

Traditionally, painkillers (analgesics) have been divided into nonopioid and opioid analgesics. The term "opioid analgesics" is derived from the fact that the first drugs in this class were found in opium (the dried sap of the opium poppy). Opioid analgesics are discussed in Sect. 2.2. Nonopioid analgesics include different drugs with different mechanisms of action and ADRs. (The prefix "non-" in "nonopioid" merely implies that they are *not* derived from opium.) In the group of nonopioid analgesics, ibuprofen, paracetamol (acetaminophen), and metamizole (dipyrone) are the most important drugs, which

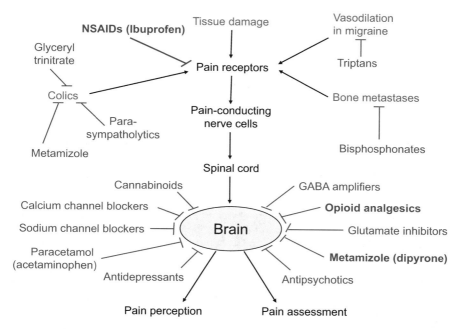

Fig. 2.1 How does pain arise, and how can it be treated? Traditionally, analgesics are divided into two classes: opioid analgesics and nonopioid analgesics. The latter group includes ibuprofen, paracetamol, and metamizole (see Fig. 2.2). Ibuprofen is the prototypical representative of the nonsteroidal anti-inflammatory drugs (NSAIDs, cyclooxygenase inhibitors). Many other drug classes can be effective for different forms of pain (for examples, see Sects. 3.3, 6.3, 8.2, 9.2, 9.4, and 11.1). Although cannabinoids are promoted in the media, their efficacy as analgesics is overrated. On the other hand, the dangers of cannabis use are underestimated (see Sects. 9.3 and 9.4). Coxibs (cyclooxygenase-2 inhibitors) are not presented here, because they can cause severe adverse drug reactions that affect the cardiovascular system

is why they are discussed in more detail in this section. Figure 2.2 compares the properties of these three drugs, and Table 2.1 provides a summary.

Many people fear that analgesics cause addiction. However, if these drugs are used with a clear indication, no such risk exists. It is not recommended to mix analgesics with caffeine. The stimulant effect of the latter can cause continuous use of mixed analgesic preparations and thus cause ADRs to the analgesics. If nonopioid analgesics are taken for a long time for (often diffuse) headaches, the pain threshold can be lowered and painkiller-induced headaches can develop. In this case, discontinuation of the drug is the solution.

Numerous other drug classes have analgesic effects. Parasympatholytics (the prototype drug is butylscopolamine) are effective against colic pain, as is glycerol trinitrate. Bisphosphonates inhibit bone resorption (see Sect. 6.3)

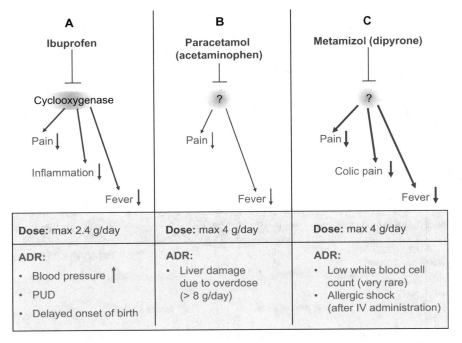

Fig. 2.2 Comparison of the properties of prototypical nonopioid analgesics: ibuprofen (a), paracetamol (acetaminophen) (b), and metamizole (dipyrone) (c). The different thicknesses of the *arrows* for the three drugs represent the differences in their maximum effects on each symptom. The maximum daily doses refer to healthy adults without kidney or liver problems. Ibuprofen, paracetamol, and metamizole are different in their effects and adverse drug reactions (ADRs), although they are all grouped in the category of nonopioid analgesics. Unlike ibuprofen, paracetamol and metamizole have no anti-inflammatory effect. Metamizole, however, has a good effect on colic pain. Ibuprofen is classified as a nonsteroidal anti-inflammatory drug (NSAID). There are also numerous other drugs in this class (e.g., diclofenac and naproxen). Paracetamol and metamizole are *not* NSAIDs

and thus relieve pain caused by bone metastases in cancer (see Sect. 11.1). Dilation of blood vessels beneath the skull causes migraines, which can be relieved by constricting the vessels with triptans.

Many drugs classified as antiepileptics (see Sect. 8.2), such as sodium and calcium channel blockers, alleviate certain forms of pain. Serotonin/norepinephrine enhancers classified as antidepressants (see Sect. 9.2) and antipsychotics used in schizophrenia (see Sect. 9.4) can relieve pain. These drug classes are particularly effective in neuropathic pain, which is difficult to treat with nonopioid and opioid analgesics, and for treatment of tumor pain (see Sect. 11.1).

Table 2.1 Overview of the most important nonopioid analgesics

Drug class	Prototype drug	Mechanisms of action	Indications	Important adverse drug reactions (ADRs) and interactions
Cyclooxygenase inhibitors (nonsteroidal anti-inflammatory drugs [NSAIDs])	Ibuprofen	Inhibition of formation of prostaglandins in the body; this mechanism mediates the desired effects and ADRs associated with ibuprofen; these drugs have analgesic, anti-inflammatory, and antipyretic effects	Mild-to-moderate pain with an inflammatory component (e.g., toothache, sports injuries, postoperative pain, acute exacerbations of chronic joint diseases, acute gouty arthritis, migraine attacks, back pain); application of these drugs should *never* exceed 2 weeks	Gastric/duodenal ulcers, reduced water and salt excretion, blood pressure increases, labor inhibition, reduced effects of blood pressure–lowering drugs, "aspirin asthma"
Pyrazolones	Metamizole (dipyrone; the only representative of this drug class with practical significance)	Unknown; this drug class is therefore designated according to its chemical structure and not its mechanism of action; it has stronger analgesic and antipyretic effects than paracetamol, relaxing effects on muscles of hollow organs, and no anti-inflammatory effect	Severe pain after surgery, high fever, colic pain, pain that does not respond to paracetamol, tumor pain; because of its different mechanism of action, metamizole can be combined with an NSAID; in some countries, metamizole is available with or without a prescription, while in others, it is not available at all	None of the typical ADRs associated with NSAIDs, no risk of peptic ulcer disease (PUD) or high blood pressure, no liver damage (unlike paracetamol); if administered intravenously (which is rare), there is a small (0.1%) risk of allergic shock; there is a small (between 1:100,000 and 1:1,000,000) risk of white blood cell depletion (agranulocytosis); therefore, regular blood cell counts are required

(continued)

Table 2.1 (continued)

Drug class	Prototype drug	Mechanisms of action	Indications	Important adverse drug reactions (ADRs) and interactions
Para-aminophenol derivatives	Paracetamol (acetaminophen; the only representative of this drug class with practical significance)	Unknown; this drug class is therefore designated according to its chemical structure and not its mechanism of action; it has weaker analgesic and antipyretic effects than metamizole, no relaxing effect on muscles of hollow organs, and no anti-inflammatory effect	Mild-to-moderate pain (especially in the absence of inflammation), tension headaches, migraines, menstrual pain; because of different mechanisms of action, paracetamol can be combined with an NSAID	None of the typical ADRs associated with NSAIDs; no risk of agranulocytosis or anaphylactic shock; there is a risk of liver damage if a daily dose of 8 g is exceeded in adults; paracetamol is given up to a maximum of 4 g/day

The three drug classes and representative drugs listed here have different properties. A common mistake in pain management is underdosing analgesics for fear of an ADR. Another common error is the use of an NSAID for too long
ADR adverse drug reaction, *NSAID* nonsteroidal anti-inflammatory drug, *PUD* peptic ulcer disease

Glutamate is an important excitatory neurotransmitter and is important for pain transmission. Therefore, glutamate inhibitors (the prototype drug is ketamine) can be used in pain therapy. Ketamine is mainly used in emergency medicine, anesthesia, and treatment of tumor pain (see Sect. 11.1). Ketamine has antidepressant effects (see Sect. 9.2).

Cannabinoids (the prototype drug is dronabinol) receive a lot of media attention. They mimic the effects of endocannabinoids produced in the body and have analgesic effects. We observe certain parallels with the endorphin/opioid receptor system (see Sect. 2.2). However, the maximum analgesic effect of cannabinoids is weaker than that of opioid analgesics.

Nonsteroidal Anti-inflammatory Drugs: Risks for the Stomach, Blood Pressure, and Kidney

Ibuprofen is one of the most widely used painkillers worldwide. Tablets, juices, and suppositories are available. Thus, it is easy to find a suitable dosage form for each patient. In adults, ibuprofen can be given up to a total daily dose of 2400 mg (2.4 g), comprising single doses of 600 mg every 6 hours or 800 mg every 8 hours. However, for fear of ADRs, ibuprofen is usually given in too low a dose (often only 200 mg), and so no pain relief is achieved. Nevertheless, ADRs can occur at this low dose. In doses of up to 400 mg per tablet, ibuprofen is a nonprescription drug in many countries.

Ibuprofen is an NSAID. However, this term is misleading because it suggests that an NSAID can be used as a long-term treatment for chronic rheumatic diseases (see Sect. 11.2). Steroids (glucocorticoids) are considered dangerous, so surely *non*steroids should be harmless! However, this is not the case. Long-term use of NSAIDs leads to severe ADRs. Therefore, this drug class should be neutrally referred to as cyclooxygenase inhibitors.

Its short duration of action (approximately 4–6 hours) makes ibuprofen suitable for treatment of acute pain. Ibuprofen prevents formation of prostaglandins by inhibiting cyclooxygenase. Prostaglandins are first messengers that regulate many bodily functions. They mediate pain, inflammation symptoms (swelling, redness, and functional impairment), and fever. Therefore, reduced prostaglandin formation caused by ibuprofen reduces pain, inflammation, and fever. All three effects are used clinically. Ibuprofen is suited to short-term treatment of toothache, bruises, sprains, back pain, tendon pain, joint pain, bone pain, and postsurgical pain. It is also effective for menstrual cramps, tension headaches, and migraines. However, ibuprofen is not effective for treatment of nerve pain (e.g., in diabetes) and colic pain in the intestines.

In most patients, short-term use of ibuprofen is not problematic, although it does increase the risk of PUD because prostaglandins are responsible for formation of the mucus that protects the stomach. However, this does not justify routine use of proton pump inhibitors in *every* treatment with ibuprofen (see Sect. 3.2).

In about 15% of all patients with allergy, treatment with ibuprofen can lead to exacerbation of allergic symptoms, known as "aspirin-induced asthma" (see Sect. 4.1). However, this term is misleading because the risk of allergic exacerbation concerns all NSAIDs, not just Aspirin® (acetylsalicylic acid, ASA).

Most ADRs associated with ibuprofen occur in long-term use, which must be avoided. Ibuprofen should not be used for longer than 2 weeks. The ADRs associated with ibuprofen in long-term treatment can be explained by reduced prostaglandin formation. In the stomach/duodenum, ulcers develop without the protective effect of prostaglandins (see Sect. 3.2). In the kidney, the vasodilating effect of prostaglandins is lost, resulting in reduced excretion of water and salt, weight gain, and increased blood pressure (see Sect. 5.1). Therefore, ibuprofen should never be used long term in patients with PUD, high blood pressure, coronary heart disease, or heart failure.

An important issue is use of ibuprofen during pregnancy. In the first two-thirds of pregnancy, ibuprofen can be used for a short time. Prostaglandins are important for labor. If a woman is constantly treated with high doses of ibuprofen toward the end of pregnancy, the onset of labor can be delayed. For safety reasons, it is recommended that ibuprofen is avoided in the third trimester and that paracetamol is used instead. Paracetamol is not problematic with respect to the onset of labor.

Diclofenac is another cyclooxygenase inhibitor on the market. Ointments containing diclofenac are popular and are used for superficial joint pain. Topical application of diclofenac is a good strategy for avoiding ADRs, but if applied too extensively (e.g., on the knee joint) and over a long period, diclofenac may cause gastrointestinal and kidney ADRs.

Problematic Coxibs

Because of the ADRs associated with NSAIDs in the stomach/duodenum, cyclooxygenase-2 (COX-2) inhibitors (coxibs; the prototype drug is etoricoxib) were developed. Unlike ibuprofen or diclofenac, these drugs do not inhibit cyclooxygenase-1 (COX-1), which is responsible for gastric protection (see Sect. 3.2). Therefore, gastric bleeding and ulcers do not occur with cyclo-oxygenase-2 inhibitors. However, the risks of strokes and myocardial infarction are so high (see Sect. 5.2) that this drug class is not an alternative to traditional cyclooxygenase inhibitors. In some countries, coxibs are not approved.

Use of Acetylsalicylic Acid for Pain Is Outdated

Historically, ASA was popular for relief of pain and inflammation. For pain, ASA is used in a single dose of 500–1000 mg (0.5–1.0 g). Unlike ibuprofen, ASA causes long-lasting inhibition of platelet clumping. Therefore, intake of ASA increases the risk of bleeding, especially in the gastrointestinal tract. To achieve a good anti-inflammatory effect, ASA must be used in daily doses of about 5 g (5 × 1 g). At these doses, ASA causes severe ADRs such as nausea, vomiting, restlessness, and ringing in the ears. Still higher doses can cause kidney failure and seizures. In children, ASA can cause life-threatening damage to the liver and brain (Reye syndrome). Therefore, ASA must not be used in infants, toddlers, or schoolchildren. Because ASA is less tolerable than ibuprofen, this drug should no longer be used for relief of pain and inflammation. In low doses (about 100 mg/day), ASA is used for secondary prevention of heart attacks and strokes (see Sect. 5.2). At this low dose, ASA has neither analgesic nor anti-inflammatory effects.

Paracetamol: Toxic for the Liver

Although paracetamol (acetaminophen) is classified as a nonopioid analgesic, there are major differences between this drug and ibuprofen or metamizole (Fig. 2.2). Ibuprofen and paracetamol have analgesic and antipyretic effects. However, paracetamol does *not* have an anti-inflammatory effect and is not as effective as ibuprofen for treatment of pain with an inflammatory component (e.g., toothache, bruises, sprains, or tendonitis). Therefore, in many cases, its analgesic effect is weaker than that of ibuprofen. For this reason, paracetamol is mainly used for mild pain and as an alternative to ibuprofen when the latter is not an option because of ADRs. The mechanism of action of paracetamol is not known. Because of its lack of effect on labor, paracetamol is considered the painkiller of choice in pregnancy.

Paracetamol is available as tablets, juices, drops, suppositories, and injection solutions, and so a suitable dosage form can be found for each patient and age group. In adults, paracetamol may be given in doses of 0.5–1.0 g

(500–1000 mg) up to four times daily. The total daily dose *must not* exceed 4 g. However, underdosing (and thus ineffectiveness) of paracetamol is much more common than overdosing.

Paracetamol is well tolerated. Unlike ibuprofen, paracetamol does not cause stomach/duodenal ulcers and does not increase blood pressure. Thus, paracetamol is a good alternative to ibuprofen in patients with these conditions. Paracetamol can be used in patients with aspirin-induced asthma. Because ibuprofen and paracetamol have different mechanisms of action, combination of the two drugs is possible (Fig. 2.2).

The main risk of paracetamol is liver damage. In adults, a single ingestion of more than 8 g (i.e., just twice the maximum daily dosage used for pain relief) may be sufficient to cause acute liver failure. The liver's detoxification capacity is insufficient when large amounts of paracetamol are ingested, and so a toxic breakdown product of the drug destroys the liver.

It is a common misconception that paracetamol is less dangerous than ibuprofen. The two drugs pose different risks. In infants and young children, care must be taken with paracetamol and the exact dose must be based on body weight. Paracetamol should be avoided in patients with liver damage (e.g., caused by hepatitis C or by alcohol addiction). These patients can suffer liver poisoning with "normal" doses of paracetamol.

Liver poisoning is often recognized only when the liver is damaged. After a latency period of about 24 hours following ingestion of a paracetamol overdose, symptoms appear. Although an antidote for paracetamol poisoning (acetylcysteine) is available, it no longer helps if it is used too late. The last resort is liver transplantation.

Paracetamol is easy to obtain. Therefore, it remains a frequent cause of accidental or suicidal poisoning. The overall toxicity of paracetamol is underestimated. It is not a safe alternative to ibuprofen but a drug with a risk profile of its own.

Metamizole: Effective but Not Available Everywhere

Metamizole (dipyrone, novaminsulfone) has a specific profile of action (Fig. 2.2): it has stronger analgesic and antipyretic effects than ibuprofen and paracetamol, and it relaxes smooth muscle cells. Therefore, metamizole is suited to treatment of more severe pain and especially colic pain (i.e., pain caused by spasm of hollow organs: intestines, bile ducts, and ureters). Since metamizole has no anti-inflammatory effect, one might assume that it does not reduce inflammation-related pain such as toothache. However, this is not true, as its overall stronger analgesic effect (in comparison with ibuprofen) compensates for this deficiency.

The mechanism of action of metamizole differs from that of ibuprofen (Fig. 2.2), which is why these two drugs can be combined in cases of severe pain. As with paracetamol, the mechanism of action is not known. Metamizole has a strong analgesic effect and is well tolerated by most patients. Metamizole does not cause PUD, aspirin-induced asthma, or an increase in blood pressure (Fig. 2.2). Unlike paracetamol, metamizole does not damage the liver. Because of its overall high efficacy and tolerability, metamizole is suitable for treatment of pain in cancer patients.

Metamizole can be used as tablets, drops, suppositories, and injection solutions. Thus, a suitable dosage form can be found for each patient. In adults, metamizole is administered in doses of up to 4 g/day (4 × 1 g at 6-hour intervals). Pain management with metamizole can be well controlled. During treatment with metamizole, the urine may turn dark because a reddish-colored degradation product is formed in the liver, but this is harmless.

The most important ADR associated with metamizole is white blood cell depletion (agranulocytosis). The (very low) risk of agranulocytosis is the major reason why metamizole is not available in some countries. In other countries, metamizole is a prescription drug, and in some countries, it is available without a prescription. Metamizole is a paradigm for cultural differences in the assessment of drug risks.

How can you recognize depletion of white blood cells? White blood cells are important for the body's defense against bacterial infections. A low white blood cell count makes it easier to contract infections (e.g., in the upper respiratory tract or the skin; see Sect. 11.3). These must then be treated with appropriate antibiotics. Fungal infections (e.g., candidiasis in the mouth or genital areas) can occur and are treated with antimycotics. Fever may be absent, as metamizole has a fever-reducing effect. To be on the safe side, the doctor will regularly monitor the white blood cell count. If detected early, agranulocytosis has a good prognosis. When metamizole is discontinued, this leads to a rebound in the white blood cell count. In severe cases, the patient may be given growth factors to stimulate white blood cell proliferation. It is important to avoid metamizole in all patients who have ever had agranulocytosis.

Another rare ADR associated with metamizole is allergic shock when the drug is administered intravenously. However, this is done only in rare cases of severe pain. Slow and controlled injection of metamizole reduces the risk of this ADR. In the event of allergic shock, epinephrine (adrenaline) must be administered immediately (see Sect. 4.1).

2.3   Opioid Analgesics

Summary

When pain becomes too severe, opioid analgesics are used. Many patients fear that opioid analgesics cause addiction. However, this is not true when they are used properly in pain management. For severe pain, opioid analgesics can be combined with nonopioid analgesics. Opioid analgesics differ in their strength of action (efficacy). Tramadol has low efficacy, buprenorphine has moderate efficacy, and morphine and fentanyl have high efficacy. The main ADRs associated with opioid analgesics are constipation and a reduction in the respiratory drive. Constipation must be treated with a laxative, preferably macrogol (a water-binding laxative). Respiratory failure can lead to death.

Memo

- Opioid analgesics have many effects in the body, not just a pain-relieving effect.
- The prototypical opioid analgesics are tramadol, buprenorphine, morphine, and fentanyl.
- These analgesics differ in their efficacy: tramadol has the lowest efficacy, buprenorphine has medium efficacy, and morphine and fentanyl have high efficacy.
- The most common ADR associated with opioid analgesics is constipation.
- Constipation is treated with macrogol.
- Especially in combination with benzodiazepines, opioid analgesics can cause respiratory failure.
- Naloxone is an antidote for opioid analgesic overdose.
- When used appropriately, opioid analgesics do not cause addiction.
- Addiction occurs when opioid analgesics are prescribed for no good reason.

How Do Opioid Analgesics Work?

Opioid analgesics (the prototype drug is morphine from opium) mimic the effects of certain first messengers, called endorphins, in the body. These first messengers activate opioid receptors (see Sect. 1.4). Opioid receptors are found throughout the body, particularly in the spinal cord and brain. One of the most important effects of opioid receptors is inhibition of pain conduction in the spinal cord and pain perception in the brain, resulting in pain relief. Endorphins are released during severe injuries and cause some pain relief from within the body itself. However, since endorphins are broken down quickly in the body, they cannot be used as drugs. Opioid analgesics act like endorphins but penetrate the brain more easily and are not broken down as quickly.

Opioid receptors mediate many other effects in the body, which may be desirable or undesirable, depending on the situation. Figure 2.3 provides an overview of the most important effects mediated by opioid receptors and shows the extent to which representative opioid analgesics elicit these effects. Table 2.2 provides an overview of the effects of opioid analgesics.

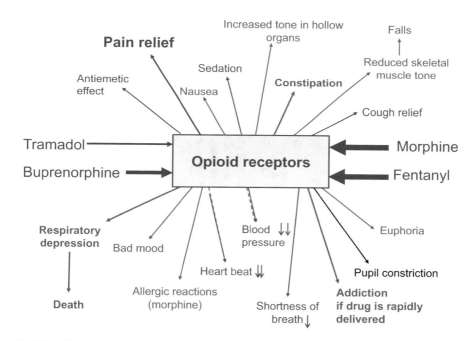

Fig. 2.3 The many effects of opioid analgesics. The different thicknesses of the *arrows* for tramadol, buprenorphine, morphine, and fentanyl represent the differences in their maximum analgesic (pain-relieving) effects. Tramadol is less pain relieving than buprenorphine, and buprenorphine is less pain relieving than morphine and fentanyl. Opioid analgesics have numerous other effects that may be desirable or undesirable, depending on the situation. When opioid analgesics are used correctly for the right indication (severe pain), the risk of addiction to them is much smaller than is commonly assumed. In contrast, the risk of addiction to opioid analgesics is high in the absence of pain and with rapid penetration of the drug into the brain. The most frequent cause of death in treatment with opioid analgesics and in abuse of opioid analgesics is respiratory arrest. Constipation usually occurs shortly after the start of treatment with opioid analgesics and can be treated with macrogol (see Table 2.2 and Sect. 3.3)

Table 2.2 Overview of representative opioid analgesics

Drug class	Prototype drug	Mechanisms of action	Indications	Important adverse drug reactions (ADRs) and interactions
Weak opioid analgesics	Tramadol	Weakest analgesic effect of all opioid analgesics; has additional mechanisms of action besides an opioid-like effect	Weak to moderate pain; often used as an alternative to ibuprofen, paracetamol or metamizole; use of combinations is possible	Risk of serotonin syndrome, hallucinations, seizures, fatigue, constipation, dyspnea, dysphagia; degraded in the liver; if combined with other drugs that are also degraded in the liver, the effects of these drugs may be amplified
Moderate opioid analgesics	Buprenorphine	Mechanism of action like that of morphine but overall lower efficacy than morphine	Severe pain that cannot be adequately controlled by tramadol but does not yet require use of morphine or fentanyl	Like those of morphine and fentanyl but weaker overall effects; with skin patches, less constipation and less respiratory depression

Drug class	Prototype drug	Mechanisms of action	Indications	Important adverse drug reactions (ADRs) and interactions
Strong opioid analgesics	Morphine	Gold standard of this drug class; has strong analgesic, sedative, antitussive, and respiratory depressant effects on opioid receptors	Severe and most severe pain (e.g., tumor pain and crushing pain in myocardial infarction); shortness of breath in pulmonary edema; used when buprenorphine no longer has sufficient effects	Initially vomiting, later inhibitory effect on vomiting; mood swings (mostly depressive mood, only rarely euphoria); inhibition of the respiratory drive; pupil constriction; constipation (must be treated with macrogol!); in the case of a wet cough, the antitussive effect causes accumulation of mucus in the lungs and increased risk of infection; drop in blood pressure
	Fentanyl	Mechanism of action like that of morphine, with similar efficacy; different dosage forms for different types of pain	Severe and most severe pain; often administered in combination with other drug classes for treatment of tumor pain; skin patches for permanent treatment of pain; lozenges and nasal spray for treatment of acute pain and breakthrough pain	Like those associated with morphine but less nausea; however, stronger suppression of the respiratory drive; risk of addiction

In this table, opioid analgesics are classified according to their maximum effects (efficacy), *not* according to their potencies. Buprenorphine is more potent than morphine but has a weaker maximum effect. Widespread classification of opioid analgesics according to their potency can result in the patient being deprived of effective pain management. This is a common mistake
ADR adverse drug reaction

Use of Opioid Analgesics

Figure 2.3 shows the effects of prototypical opioid analgesics. The main difference between the individual drugs is in their maximum analgesic effects. Tramadol has only a mild analgesic effect, buprenorphine has a medium effect, and morphine and fentanyl have strong effects.

Initially, pain is usually treated with nonopioid analgesics (see Sect. 2.1). If nonopioid analgesics are not sufficient, opioid analgesics are used as an alternative or in addition. Usually, opioid therapy starts with tramadol, then buprenorphine; ultimately, morphine and fentanyl are administered. Thus, pain therapy is based on the intensity of pain. This is particularly important in treatment of pain in cancer patients (see Sect. 11.1).

Opioid analgesics are opioid receptor agonists (see Sect. 1.4). Permanent activation of these receptors in long-term treatment may lead to loss of efficacy of the corresponding drug. During long-term therapy with opioid analgesics, it may be necessary to increase the dose to achieve the same analgesic effect in the long term.

Many Effects of Opioid Analgesics

The term "opioid analgesics" emphasizes the analgesic effect of this drug class, but these drugs have other effects that may be either desirable or undesirable, depending on the situation (Fig. 2.3). The sedative effect of opioid analgesics can be used especially in treatment of severe pain in cancer patients, and it facilitates sleep. However, this implies that patients' intellectual performance is impaired, as is their ability to drive and operate machinery.

The cough-relieving effect of opioid analgesics can be used for a dry irritating cough, especially in upper respiratory tract infections. Codeine is often used for this purpose. Opioid analgesics should not be used for a wet cough, because secretions can back up in the lungs, making it easier for pneumonia to develop.

What opioid analgesics are best known for is that they can cause addiction. However, the risk of addiction is low when these drugs are used in pain patients. If, on the other hand, a person has no pain and the opioid analgesic enters the brain quickly (e.g., when heroin is injected intravenously), the risk of addiction is high. For this reason, pain therapy with opioid analgesics tries to avoid such peaks and the drugs are administered regularly (by the clock), orally (by the mouth), and gradually (by the ladder).

In pain patients, opioid analgesics often induce a depressive mood. Although at first glance this seems to be a negative effect of opioid analgesics, it is ultimately positive because (in contrast to euphoria) this counteracts misuse of these drugs.

Nausea is common at the start of treatment with opioid analgesics and can be treated with metoclopramide (see Sect. 3.1). Later, it tends to be replaced by an antiemetic effect.

The most common and most important ADR associated with opioid analgesics is constipation (see Sect. 3.3). Constipation occurs immediately after starting treatment with opioid analgesics. Therefore, constipation must be addressed, especially in long-term treatment. Constipation caused by opioid analgesics can be controlled safely with macrogol (see Sect. 3.3).

Opioid analgesics can contract smooth muscle cells in hollow organs such as bile ducts and ureters. This causes colic pain. Accordingly, opioid analgesics should not be used in cases of known biliary or kidney stone disease. For colic pain, metamizole or glycerol trinitrate (see Sect. 2.1) can be given. These drugs relax smooth muscle cells in bile ducts and ureters.

Particularly with morphine, and much less frequently with other opioid analgesics, allergy-like reactions can occur (see Sect. 4.1). This is because morphine can directly activate mast cells without involvement of antigens. However, these reactions are rarely severe. If a mast cell reaction occurs after administration of morphine, it is no problem to switch to another opioid analgesic that does not cause these mast cell reactions.

A matter of considerable practical importance is the fact that opioid analgesics reduce the tension of skeletal muscles. Consequently, patients may be less able to maintain their balance and may thus fall. The risk of falls is particularly high when elderly patients are simultaneously given benzodiazepines, which reduce muscle tone (see Sect. 8.2). This combination of drugs should therefore be avoided unless the patient has somebody permanently around who takes care of them and can prevent them from falling.

Opioid analgesics can reduce breathlessness in emergency situations such as myocardial infarction (see Sect. 5.2) or pulmonary embolism. However, the flip side is that opioid analgesics cause respiratory depression. A patient can stop breathing and suffocate without experiencing shortness of breath. This dangerous ADR is one of the most common causes of death during opioid analgesic therapy, especially when this type of drug is taken at higher doses and for longer periods. Therefore, the patient's use of the correct dosage must be monitored to avoid accidental overdoses resulting in respiratory arrest (cessation of breathing). This risk becomes greater when tumor patients take benzodiazepines in parallel with opioid analgesics.

Opioid analgesics can cause pupillary constriction. Constricted pupils, in combination with unconsciousness and inhibition of the respiratory drive, may point to opioid analgesic intoxication.

Opioid analgesics decrease the heart rate and lower blood pressure. If the heart rate and blood pressure are high, this effect is desired. If the heart rate and blood pressure are low, it is more likely to be an ADR.

Addiction to Opioid Analgesics

Euphoria is the most common cause of opioid analgesic abuse. This effect occurs when the drug enters the brain rapidly. A rapid onset of opioid analgesics can be achieved by intravenous injection. Heroin (a precursor of morphine) is used for this purpose and reaches the brain extremely quickly. Therefore, heroin has much greater addiction potential than morphine. In the meantime, fentanyl, which is used in treatment of pain, is becoming increasingly important as an addictive substance because its fat solubility causes it to enter the brain rapidly (see Sect. 1.5). To avoid addiction, opioid analgesics are not used intravenously in pain therapy, with a few exceptions (e.g., for extreme pain in myocardial infarction and extreme breathlessness in pulmonary edema).

The risk of opioid analgesic addiction depends on the initial situation the body is in. If a person has no pain, the risks of euphoria and addiction are much greater than if a patient has chronic pain from cancer. Prescribing of opioid analgesics for trivial headaches, osteoarthritis, mood disorders, unclear mental problems, or dementia increases the risk of addiction.

In opioid analgesic addiction, the purpose of one's life revolves around obtaining and taking opioid analgesics. Once the level of opioid analgesics in the body drops, psychological withdrawal symptoms (such as anxiety, nightmares, depression, and aggression) and physical withdrawal symptoms (such as shivering ["cold turkey"], restlessness, and palpitations) develop. Such a situation rarely occurs in pain therapy.

An acute life-threatening danger is respiratory arrest caused by administration of high doses of opioid analgesics. In the event of respiratory arrest, an emergency doctor must inject the antidote naloxone. It acts as an antagonist, displacing the opioid analgesics from their receptors (see Sect. 1.4), and breathing resumes. At the same time, however, withdrawal symptoms occur. Naloxone has a rapid onset of action but a short duration of action. It is therefore well suited to treatment of emergency situations but not to long-term treatment.

Addiction to opioid analgesics can be treated in two ways. One way is for the patient to go through withdrawal, with all of the unpleasant accompanying symptoms. The withdrawal symptoms can be thought of as biofeedback that makes the patient realize the damage they have done to themselves. It is possible to mitigate the withdrawal symptoms with clonidine. After going through withdrawal, the patient must consistently stay away from opioid analgesics, otherwise they will immediately slip back into addiction. This can be avoided by long-term treatment with naltrexone. Naltrexone acts as an antagonist, occupying the opioid receptors and thus preventing opioid analgesics from producing effects when they are taken (see Sect. 1.4). Unlike naloxone, naltrexone has a long duration of action.

The second option for treating opioid analgesic addiction is substitution with long-acting opioid analgesics. This substitution is usually done with methadone. It is dispensed at official locations and must be taken on-site to prevent the methadone from being resold. Oral administration of methadone prevents withdrawal symptoms, and euphoria (a feeling of happiness) is absent because of the slow onset of the drug's action in the brain. Through these substitution programs, many opioid analgesic addicts can be reintegrated into society, and crime and prostitution, which are often coupled with opioid analgesic addiction, can be avoided.

Tramadol: Popular and Overrated

Tramadol is popular in several countries. However, the analgesic effect of tramadol is overrated. It is only 10% of the maximum effect of morphine, and use of tramadol leads to patients with severe pain being underserved.

In addition, it is doubtful whether tramadol acts only through opioid receptors. Other mechanisms of action are involved, such as inhibition of serotonin reuptake into nerve cells (see Sect. 9.2). This assumption is supported by the fact that tramadol, like serotonin reuptake inhibitors, can cause serotonin syndrome (nausea, vomiting, high blood pressure, headaches, seizures, tremors, and hallucinations).

Tramadol can relieve mild-to-moderate pain. Because of its short duration of action (1–3 hours), it is suitable for acute pain and can be used as an alternative to the nonopioid analgesics ibuprofen, paracetamol, and metamizole if they are ineffective or ADRs prevent their administration (see Sect. 2.1).

Buprenorphine: Less Effective Than Morphine

If tramadol does not provide sufficient pain relief, the next stage of pain treatment is buprenorphine. Buprenorphine can be given as a capsule under the tongue or is applied to the skin as a patch because it is not well absorbed into the body when given orally. Buprenorphine has a long duration of action, so it is well suited to long-term treatment of severe pain. However, the maximum effect of buprenorphine is weaker than that of morphine and fentanyl. This applies to both desired effects and ADRs.

Morphine: The Gold Standard

Morphine is the gold standard of opioid analgesics—in other words, all opioid analgesics are compared with morphine. Morphine has more pronounced effects than buprenorphine in terms of both desired effects and ADRs.

When administered intravenously, morphine may induce mast cell activation and should therefore be reserved for special emergency situations. This mast cell activation does not play a role when morphine is given orally. For long-term therapy, morphine has too short a duration of action (about 4 hours). Therefore, special sustained-release forms of morphine and morphine derivatives (the prototype drug is hydromorphone), with a much longer duration of action (8–12 hours), are used. These dosage forms are suited to long-term treatment of pain, as the aim is to prevent pain from occurring in the first place.

A common mistake is to combine a strong opioid analgesic, such as morphine, with buprenorphine. Instead of enhancing the effect, this combination lowers the effect of the strong opioid analgesic to the level of the less effective opioid analgesic. If the effect of morphine is insufficient, it makes much more sense to increase the morphine dose to compensate for the loss of the effect due to habituation.

Fentanyl: Versatile but Risky

Fentanyl has a maximum effect comparable to that of morphine but is more fat soluble than morphine. Thus, fentanyl penetrates the brain and relieves pain more quickly than morphine. This property of fentanyl can be used to provide rapid relief in acute pain situations. Fentanyl can be used in the form of lozenges or nasal spray for acute pain. However, there have been cases of people mistaking xylometazoline or naphazoline decongestant nasal drops (which are intended for use in the common cold but can have psychoactive effects) for fentanyl and misusing them. It is essential to ensure that this does not occur, as it can lead to serious ADRs and death.

Fentanyl is suitable not only for acute treatment of pain but also for long-term treatment of pain. For this purpose, a fentanyl skin patch is applied. From this depot, fentanyl is slowly absorbed into the body. Unfortunately, however, fentanyl patches are sometimes misused. They are sometimes pulled off the skin of pain patients by opioid analgesic addicts, who open the patches and swallow the contents of the patch by mouth. Because of its good fat solubility, the fentanyl is rapidly absorbed into the body and thus into the brain, and this leads to the feeling of euphoria desired by addicted individuals. To counteract misuse of fentanyl patches and interruption of pain therapy in patients, fentanyl patches should be applied only to parts of the body that will be covered by clothes (i.e., not on the neck or forearm; see Fig. 2.3).

3

Drugs for Gastrointestinal Disorders

Abstract Gastroesophageal reflux disease is caused by reflux of acid into the esophagus. Elimination of its causes is crucial in the treatment of gastroesophageal reflux disease. It can be effectively treated with proton pump inhibitors. However, you should be cautious with their long-term use. The most important cause of peptic ulcer disease is an infection with the bacterium *Helicobacter pylori*. It can be treated with certain antibiotics and proton pump inhibitors. Long-term use of nonsteroidal anti-inflammatory drugs is another cause of peptic ulcer disease. Constipation is a result of a low-fiber diet, lack of exercise, and long-term use of laxatives. In addition, certain drugs can cause constipation. The decisive factor in treatment of constipation is elimination of its causes. Laxatives should be used only on a short-term basis. Diarrhea is usually caused by viruses and is treated by adequate replacement of water and salts. Loperamide can be used on a short-term basis. It reduces the stool frequency.

3.1 Gastroesophageal Reflux Disease

Summary

Gastroesophageal reflux disease (GERD) is common. GERD must be treated because otherwise esophageal ulcers develop, which can lead to bleeding or esophageal cancer. Treatment focuses on elimination of causes. Self-treatment with antacids and H_2 receptor blockers is not recommended, because their effectiveness is inadequate and they may delay proper diagnosis. GERD is most effectively treated with proton pump inhibitors (PPIs). However, be warned against long-term therapy with PPIs, as it can lead to adverse drug reactions (ADRs) such as vitamin B_{12} and calcium deficiencies.

Memo

- Lifestyle measures can prevent GERD in many cases.
- Avoid late and fatty meals in combination with alcohol.
- GERD must be treated because otherwise it can lead to dangerous secondary diseases.
- Numerous drug classes—including bisphosphonates, parasympatholytic drugs, and oral contraceptives—can exacerbate GERD.
- Antacids and H_2 receptor blockers have only limited efficacy in treating GERD.
- PPIs are the most important and effective drug class used for treating GERD.
- Long-term treatment with PPIs can lead to deficiencies of vitamin B_{12}, calcium, and iron.
- Metoclopramide (MCP) normalizes the motility of the gastrointestinal tract in GERD, nausea, and vomiting.
- In infants and young children, metoclopramide may cause involuntary movements (dyskinesia).

How Does Gastroesophageal Reflux Disease Develop?

GERD is one of the most common reasons for consultations with doctors and pharmacists. Heartburn is the leading symptom of GERD and is caused by reflux of acidic stomach contents into the esophagus. The esophagus transports food and drink from the mouth into the stomach. Hence, it must contract and relax in an orderly manner. In the stomach, gastric acid acts on foods. However, stomach acid is a double-edged sword: on the one hand, it is important for digestion; on the other hand, it can erode the esophagus when it flows back the stomach entrance. Swallowing difficulties may occur.

Figure 3.1 shows the development of GERD. The entrance to the stomach (cardia) plays a key role in this process. All factors leading to slackening of the cardia promote development of GERD. Therefore, in treatment of GERD, it is important to eliminate all slackening factors. You can best find out for yourself which factors are most harmful to you and avoid them.

A simple measure to avoid GERD during the night is sleeping on your back with your head elevated. Avoid lying flat on your back or stomach. If you think of GERD as minor discomfort and do not pay further attention to it, further problems may arise, such as coughing, hoarseness, bronchitis, laryngitis, sinusitis, tooth decay, and sleep disorders. If GERD is left untreated, esophagitis can develop. If esophagitis goes untreated, narrowing (strictures), bleeding, and (in the worst case) esophageal cancer can develop. So, take GERD seriously and don't try self-treatment for too long. You will lose precious time. The best way to find out what is going on in your esophagus is to

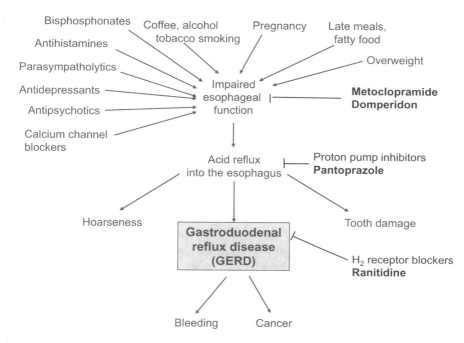

Fig. 3.1 How does gastroesophageal reflux disease (GERD) develop, and how is it treated? Numerous drug classes can promote GERD. GERD can cause dental damage and hoarseness. A major problem is uncritical long-term use of proton pump inhibitors (PPIs). Severe adverse drug reactions (ADRs; see the text) can occur if PPIs are taken for years. Of particular importance in treatment of GERD is avoidance of various trigger factors. Self-treatment with H_2 receptor blockers is problematic because it is insufficient and delays medical diagnosis

have esophagoscopy. This can be done on an outpatient basis under sedation (e.g., with the benzodiazepine midazolam; see Sect. 8.2).

Proton Pumps in the Stomach Are the Most Important Target for Treatment of Gastroesophageal Reflux Disease

Without acid, GERD does not occur. Therefore, it is important to understand how stomach acid formation works. Stomach acid is hydrochloric acid. Parietal cells in the lining of the stomach have pumps that shovel hydrochloric acid out of the cells into the stomach. These proton pumps are the main target for GERD drugs called proton pump inhibitors (PPIs).

Proton pumps are activated by different first messengers such as histamine. The effects of histamine on gastric acid production are mediated by the histamine H_2 receptor. Therefore, H_2 receptor antagonists (H_2 receptor blockers) can inhibit acid formation but only partially.

What Are the Causes of Gastroesophageal Reflux Disease?

Figure 3.1 shows some causes of GERD. Eliminating the causes is the key to successful treatment. Common causes of GERD are obesity or pregnancy. In obesity, abdominal fat presses on the stomach inlet; in pregnancy, the fetus presses on the stomach inlet. Accordingly, weight loss is the key to preventing GERD in obesity. Heartburn that is due to pregnancy stops with birth. Dietary habits and stimulants play important roles in triggering GERD. Fatty foods and late meals promote development of GERD, as does consumption of strong coffee, alcohol, and tobacco products.

Several drugs can relax the entrance to the stomach and promote GERD by facilitating reflux of acid into the esophagus. These include parasympatholytics (muscarinic receptor antagonists such as biperiden; see Sect. 8.1), drugs used to treat spasms in the gastrointestinal tract and uterus (e.g., butylscopolamine; see Sect. 3.3), glycerol trinitrate (used for treatment of angina pectoris), theophylline (used for treatment of chronic obstructive pulmonary disease [COPD]; see Sect. 4.2), calcium channel blockers (used for treatment of high blood pressure; see Sect. 5.1), phosphodiesterase type 5 (PDE5) inhibitors (used for erectile dysfunction; see Sect. 7.2), and estrogen derivatives (used as oral contraceptives or hormone replacement therapy; see Sect. 7.1). Other drugs that can cause GERD include certain antipsychotics (e.g., promethazine; see Sect. 9.4), high-dose antihistamines (e.g., clemastine; see Sect. 4.1), and certain antidepressants (e.g., amitriptyline; see Sect. 9.2). It is important to tell your doctor or pharmacist which drugs you are taking if you have GERD.

Bisphosphonates pose a particular risk of causing esophageal damage. This drug class is used to treat osteoporosis (see Sect. 6.3). It is important that you take bisphosphonates in the morning on an empty stomach with a glass of water and that you do not lie down again afterward; otherwise, you may develop severe esophageal burns with associated symptoms.

What Options Do You Have for Self-Treatment?

As explained above, the key to the treatment of GERD is elimination of its causes. If these measures are not sufficient, it is necessary to use drug therapy. Several drugs for treatment of GERD are available without a prescription in many countries. These include antacids, H_2 receptor blockers, and PPIs. Table 3.1 summarizes important drug classes used for treatment of

Table 3.1 Overview of the most important drug classes used for treatment of gastro-esophageal disease (GERD)

Drug class	Prototype drug	Mechanisms of action	Indications	Important adverse drug reactions (ADRs) and interactions
Antacids	Aluminum hydroxide	Short-term neutralization of stomach acid	Short-term self-treatment of GERD; not to be used for long-term treatment	Constipation; risk of delayed diagnosis of GERD
	Magnesium hydroxide	Short-term neutralization of stomach acid	Short-term self-treatment of GERD; not to be used for long-term treatment	Diarrhea; risk of delayed diagnosis of GERD
H_2 receptor blockers	Rani**tidine**	Short-term inhibition of stomach acid formation stimulated by histamine	Short-term self-treatment of GERD; not to be used for long-term treatment; widely used for "stress ulcer prophylaxis" in hospitals (but unproven efficacy)	Risk of delayed diagnosis of GERD
Prokinetics	Metoclopramide (MCP)	Normalization of movements in the gastrointestinal tract from "bottom up" to "top down"	Nausea and feeling of fullness associated with GERD and diarrhea; short-term use in adolescents and adults (*not* in infants and young children)	Involuntary (harmless but socially irritating) muscle twitching in the face and neck (acute dystonia), for which an antidote (biperiden) is available

(continued)

Table 3.1 (continued)

Drug class	Prototype drug	Mechanisms of action	Indications	Important adverse drug reactions (ADRs) and interactions
Proton pump inhibitors (PPIs)	Panto**prazole**	Long-term and complete inhibition of stomach acid formation by proton pump inhibition	Short-term self-treatment of GERD; short- and long-term medical treatment of GERD	Decreased absorption of iron, magnesium, calcium, and vitamin B_{12} into the body, which may result in corresponding deficiencies; rebound acid secretion in the event of sudden discontinuation after long-term therapy; nausea, vomiting, constipation, diarrhea; various long-term risks (e.g., dementia, kidney damage, infections)

Drug-specific word stems are shown in bold text. Because of the common focus on brand-names, inadvertent double prescribing of PPIs occurs frequently. Look for the suffix "_prazole" in the international nonproprietary names (INNs) of PPIs to avoid double prescribing

ADR adverse drug reaction, *GERD* gastroesophageal reflux disease, *INN* international nonproprietary name, *MCP* metoclopramide, *PPI* proton pump inhibitor

GERD. Self-treatment for GERD should only be carried out in the short term since it is often insufficient and masks the severity of the disease.

In the past, antacids were the drugs used most often for GERD. They buffer the stomach acid for a short time. Magnesium-containing antacids can cause diarrhea. Aluminum-containing antacids can cause constipation. Some antacids contain both magnesium and aluminum. These antacids hardly affect bowel movements and are the most tolerable. Be sure to pay attention to the composition of antacids. The main problem with use of antacids for GERD is their insufficient effectiveness.

H₂ Receptor Blockers

As an alternative to antacids, H_2 receptor blockers are often used. They were the first effective drug class to become available for treatment of GERD and peptic ulcer disease (PUD). However, H_2 receptor blockers are an example of how quickly medical progress can become obsolete. This is because histamine is merely one of several activators of acid formation. In contrast, the proton pump represents the common end point of all pathways leading to acid formation. Therefore, PPIs are much more effective against GERD than H_2 receptor blockers.

H_2 receptor blockers are still used because doctors and pharmacists have grown up with this principle of action. All drugs in this class can be recognized by the drug class–specific suffix "_tidine" in these drugs' international nonproprietary names (INNs). One advantage of H_2 receptor blockers is that they cause hardly any ADRs. H_2 receptor blockers are routinely used in many hospitals for "stomach protection". This use is unnecessary.

Self-Medication with Proton Pump Inhibitors

Long-term treatment of GERD with H_2 receptor blockers is not advisable because they are not effective enough. They have largely been replaced by PPIs in self-treatment. In many countries, you can buy PPIs over the counter.

Short-term treatment of GERD with a PPI (for a maximum 3–5 days) on your own is justifiable. However, if the symptoms do not disappear within that time, you should consult your doctor. A special feature of PPIs is that they permanently inhibit proton pumps. After treatment with this type of drug, the body must remake new proton pumps. After you take a PPI once (in the morning), it takes 2 days for the effect to be completely reversed.

How Your Doctor Treats Gastroesophageal Reflux Disease

Long-term treatment of GERD belongs in the hands of your doctor because it requires comprehensive diagnosis. As a rule, your doctor will treat GERD with a PPI. Worldwide, PPIs are among the most frequently prescribed drugs. You can recognize the name of a PPI by the typical suffix "_prazole" in its INN. This is important because the brand-names of PPIs do not have this typical suffix. This makes it too easy for PPIs to be prescribed twice by different doctors because treatment and prophylaxis (prevention) of "stress" and "stomach protection" (see Sect. 5.3) play important psychological roles in many doctors' offices: with a PPI pill every morning, you can (supposedly) do something "good" for yourself and protect yourself from the challenges of life!

Avoid accidental double prescribing of PPIs by looking for the typical suffix "_prazole" in the INN on the drug package. The differences between the individual drugs are only small.

Your doctor will usually prescribe a standard PPI dose (e.g., 40 mg of pantoprazole) for 4–8 weeks. The PPI is taken about 30 minutes before breakfast. In most cases, the symptoms improve within a week. The healing of esophageal changes (inflammation and bleeding) should be checked with esophagoscopy.

Without eliminating causative factors, the rate of GERD recurrence GERD is high. "Convenient" treatment of GERD with PPIs is just an attempt to neglect the need to eliminate its causes. As a result of this convenience and the chronic nature of GERD, PPIs are often prescribed for years or sometimes even for decades without a thought about the consequences.

"Stomach Protection" with a Proton Pump Inhibitor During Treatment with Acetylsalicylic Acid or Clopidogrel

One reason for use of PPIs is supposed "stomach protection" during treatment with drugs that prevent coronary heart disease or strokes. These include clopidogrel and low-dose acetylsalicylic acid (ASA; see Sect. 5.2). While these drugs can indeed cause bleeding in the gastrointestinal tract, routine prescribing of a PPI for every patient using them is not justified.

If a patient with a history of coronary heart disease or a stroke must take clopidogrel or ASA to prevent another event, the first step is to get along without "stomach protection" from a PPI. In most cases, this is possible. PPIs are frequently given as "stomach protection" in the hospital. No benefit from this type of precautionary PPI treatment has been demonstrated. Rather, this use of PPIs is far too often the starting point for unnecessary prescribing of PPIs after hospitalization.

It is worth trying to discontinue PPI use after many years. However, this must be done gradually over a period of a few weeks with careful observation of any symptoms. In many cases, you and your doctor will find that the PPI is not necessary and that you suddenly feel better because the ADRs of the PPI have disappeared.

However, if continuous PPI therapy for years is indicated, an attempt should be made to halve the drug dose. The patient either takes half a standard dose (e.g., 20 mg of pantoprazole) daily or takes a full dose (40 mg) every other day. Both approaches are possible because PPIs inhibit proton pumps long term. Be sure to avoid suddenly stopping a PPI after long-term use. This can lead to stomach acidity and severe GERD.

What Are the Risks of Taking a Proton Pump Inhibitor for Many Years?

If you take a PPI for a long time, you reduce the risk of GERD and esophageal disease, on the one hand, but on the other hand, you change the stomach function. The stomach contents are no longer acidic; rather, they are alkaline. Your doctor will need to check your blood count regularly, as well as your levels of vitamin B_{12}, iron, and calcium. PPI use can reduce absorption of vitamin B_{12}, iron, and calcium into the body, causing anemia, nerve damage, and osteoporosis (see Sect. 6.3). For this reason, regular checkups with a neurologist and bone density measurements must be carried out. To avoid ADRs associated with PPIs, a diet rich in iron, calcium, and vitamin B_{12} is recommended.

If you are found to have vitamin B_{12} deficiency, your doctor will need to inject you with this vitamin intravenously. It is controversial as to how much PPI use increases the incidence rates of stomach infections with certain bacteria, pneumonia, dementia, chronic kidney disease, and gastric cancer. Uncertainty in assessment of these potential risks is an argument for limiting treatment with a PPI to 4–8 weeks, if possible.

PPIs can cause ADRs such as headaches, dizziness, nausea, vomiting, diarrhea, and constipation. If you are taking a PPI and you experience any of these symptoms, you must consider the PPI as the likely cause, no matter whether you are taking it on prescription or as self-medication.

The change in the stomach function caused by PPIs can lead to a delay in absorption of certain drugs such as antimycotics and drugs used to treat human immunodeficiency virus (HIV). Finally, some PPIs inhibit drug breakdown in the liver, which can lead to drug interactions. PPIs are drugs, not "dietary supplements". Unfortunately, this distinction is often forgotten. Therefore, every use of a PPI should be critically reviewed to avoid misuse and associated ADRs.

When Is Metoclopramide Used?

In some patients with GERD, the cause of the discomfort is not only relaxation of the entrance to the stomach but also disturbed movement of the esophagus and stomach: the normal movements "from top to bottom" are reversed "from bottom to top". These changes in motility manifest themselves as nausea, a feeling of fullness, and vomiting. They occur in gastrointestinal infections (see Sect. 3.3).

To treat a feeling of fullness, nausea, and vomiting, prokinetics such as metoclopramide can be used. They reverse the disturbed movements in the gastrointestinal tract in the direction "from top to bottom" and thus eliminate the symptoms.

Metoclopramide should be used only on a short-term basis for acute symptoms. In the event of an overdose (especially in children), it can cause involuntary movements of the muscles of the face and neck. These movement disorders (acute dystonia) are only temporary and harmless, but they are irritating and socially awkward for the affected patient. If treatment of dyskinesia becomes necessary, your doctor can prescribe biperiden, which is a muscarinic receptor antagonist (also known as a parasympatholytic; see Sect. 8.1). However, this is only necessary in exceptional cases.

3.2   Peptic Ulcer Disease

Summary

PUD is caused by an imbalance of protective and damaging factors. The most important damaging factor is an infection with the bacterium *Helicobacter pylori*. Accordingly, antibiotics play an important role in treatment. An increased concentration of gastric acid has a damaging effect. Therefore, PPIs are used for treatment of PUD. Long-term treatment with glucocorticoids and nonsteroidal anti-inflammatory drugs (NSAIDs) promotes development of PUD. This requires consideration of alternative treatment options. Long-term treatment of coronary heart disease with low-dose ASA or clopidogrel does not have to be routinely accompanied by concomitant PPI treatment.

Memo

- The most important cause of PUD is an infection with the bacterium *Helicobacter pylori.*
- Bacterially caused PUD can be cured with two antibiotics and a PPI.
- Long-term therapy with an NSAID increases the risk of PUD.
- "Stomach protection" with prostaglandins is outdated because they cause considerable ADRs.
- Long-term therapy with glucocorticoids can promote PUD.
- "Stomach protection" with a PPI during long-term therapy with low-dose ASA must be well justified to outweigh the ADRs caused by PPIs.

How Does Peptic Ulcer Disease Develop, and How Is It Treated?

PUD is characterized by profound damage to the gastrointestinal mucosa. Bleeding can occur and, in the worst case, the ulcer can develop into cancer. Therefore, PUD must be treated. The symptoms of PUD differ from those of GERD (see Sect. 3.1). Upper abdominal pain occurring approximately 1–3 hours after eating is typical. This pain is mitigated by food intake.

PUD results from an imbalance between protective and damaging factors. Figure 3.2 shows the development of PUD and the therapeutic options. Protective factors include avoidance of stress, good mucosal blood flow, and adequate mucus production. Accordingly, stress, poor mucosal blood flow, and insufficient mucus secretion promote ulceration. Another damaging factor is increased formation of gastric acid. An infection with the bacterium

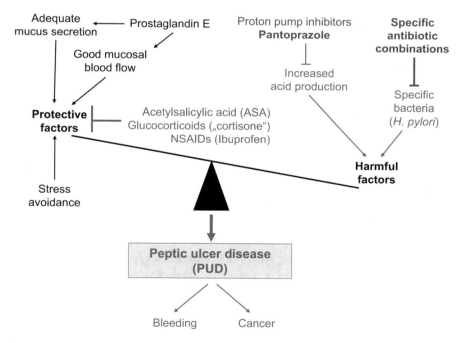

Fig. 3.2 How does peptic ulcer disease (PUD) develop, and how is it treated? This disease is a prime example of a disturbance in the balance (homeostasis) between protective and damaging factors. The goal is to strengthen protective factors and to weaken or eliminate harmful factors. Other examples of diseases with disturbed homeostasis are shown in the form of a scale in Figs. 3.3, 6.3, 8.1, 8.2, 10.1, and 11.3. Of particular importance for PUD is avoidance of causative drugs and treatment with specific antibiotic combinations

Helicobacter pylori, which is adapted to the specific conditions in the stomach, is a common cause of PUD. The bacterium triggers chronic inflammation, which can lead to an ulcer and ultimately to cancer.

PUD is diagnosed by endoscopy of the stomach and duodenum. During this process, small tissue samples are removed to test for the presence of *Helicobacter pylori*. The bacterium is detected in more than 70% of all stomach ulcers and in more than 90% of all duodenal ulcers.

It took a long time before it was accepted that an infection with the bacterium *Helicobacter pylori* is a common cause of PUD. Once the bacterium has been detected, the "treat once successfully" principle is applied. Table 3.2 summarizes the properties of the most important drugs for treatment of PUD.

In one type of therapy, a PPI (the prototype drug is pantoprazole) is combined with the two antibiotics amoxicillin (an aminopenicillin) and clarithromycin (a macrolide antibiotic). The drugs are taken orally over a period of 7–14 days. The two antibiotics are usually well tolerated. With amoxicillin, diarrhea (due to disturbance of the intestinal microbiome) is the most common ADR (see Sect. 11.3). Clarithromycin inhibits degradation of certain other drugs and thus may enhance the effects of the lipid-lowering drug simvastatin (see Sect. 5.2) and the anticoagulant warfarin (see Sect. 5.2). Therefore, before starting therapy with clarithromycin, it is essential to check your medication and reduce the doses of other drugs you take, if necessary.

In another type of therapy, a PPI is combined with clarithromycin and metronidazole. Metronidazole mainly causes taste disturbances and burning of the tongue and mouth, but it can also cause alcohol intolerance, headaches, balance disorders, and nerve tingling (polyneuropathy). As a precaution, metronidazole should not be used in pregnant women or nursing mothers. Another important safety measure is not to continue treatment with metronidazole for more than 2 weeks. The success of the treatment is checked by endoscopy.

In some cases, *Helicobacter pylori* is resistant to the antibiotics discussed above. PUD then persists despite treatment. In these cases, other specific antibiotics can be used.

How Does Nonsteroidal Anti-inflammatory Drug Treatment Cause Peptic Ulcer Disease?

To understand how NSAIDs cause PUD, it is necessary to consider, once again, the balance between protective and damaging factors. Two important factors that protect the stomach are good mucosal blood flow and adequate

Table 3.2 Overview of the most important antibiotics used for treatment of peptic ulcer disease (PUD)

Drug class	Prototype drug	Mechanisms of action	Indications	Important adverse drug reactions (ADRs) and interactions
Aminopenicillins	**Amoxicillin**	Inhibition of cell wall formation in *Helicobacter pylori*; hence, killing of these bacteria	Gastric/duodenal ulcer with proven *Helicobacter pylori* infection	Allergies (wheals in 1–10% of all patients, allergic shock in 1 in 100,000 patients); diarrhea; in rare cases, overgrowth of dangerous bacteria in the intestinal microbiome (pseudomembranous enterocolitis)
Macrolides	Clarithromycin	Inhibition of protein formation in *Helicobacter pylori*; hence, slowing of bacterial growth	Gastric/duodenal ulcer with proven *Helicobacter pylori* infection	Nausea, vomiting, diarrhea; inhibition of liver enzymes, leading to increased (undesired) effects of various drugs such as ciclosporin (an immunosuppressant), valproic acid (an antiepileptic), warfarin (an anticoagulant), and simvastatin (a lipid-lowering drug)
Nitroimidazoles	Metronidazole	Binding to genetic material (DNA [deoxyribonucleic acid]) of *Helicobacter pylori*; hence, killing of these bacteria	Gastric/duodenal ulcer with proven *Helicobacter pylori* infection; alternative to amoxicillin in the event of penicillin allergy	Metallic taste, mouth and tongue inflammation, alcohol intolerance, headaches, nerve tingling, balance disorders

Drug-specific word stems are shown in bold text. Proton pump inhibitors (PPIs) are discussed in Sect. 3.1. The antibiotics listed here are prescription only and must never be taken without medical consultation. The main danger is development of resistance to antibiotics, which can have far-reaching consequences (see Sect. 11.3)

ADR adverse drug reaction, *DNA* deoxyribonucleic acid, *PPI* proton pump inhibitor, *PUD* peptic ulcer disease

mucus production. These two factors are enhanced by the first messenger prostaglandin E. However, prostaglandin E is a double-edged sword because it causes fever, pain, and symptoms of inflammation (see Sects. 2.1 and 11.2).

NSAIDs inhibit formation of prostaglandin E, which is why they are so commonly used in treatment of pain, inflammation, and fever (see Sect. 2.1). In most cases, short-term use of an NSAID is not problematic for gastric function. However, treatment with an NSAID should not be continued for longer than 2 weeks, as the risk of PUD increases. If long-term treatment is required, three options are available:

1. Dose reduction of the NSAID.
2. Addition of a PPI to the NSAID. In this case, ADRs associated with long-term PPI treatment must be considered (see Sect. 3.1).
3. A switch to another analgesic drug, such as metamizole, paracetamol, or tramadol (see Sects. 2.1 and 2.2). These drugs pose no risk of PUD.

Two other alternatives are *not* recommended:

1. In some preparations, an NSAID is combined with a prostaglandin E_2 derivative (the prototype drug is misoprostol) as "stomach protection". However, misoprostol is ineffective and poorly tolerated. It can cause headaches, nausea, vomiting, diarrhea, and intestinal cramps. It can cause uterine cramps in women, and pregnant women are at risk of spontaneous abortion. In some countries without legal abortion, misoprostol is used to terminate pregnancies via this effect.
2. Certain drugs (known as coxibs) have anti-inflammatory and analgesic effects but pose a low risk of PUD. However, coxibs (the prototype drug is etoricoxib) have a high risk of promoting cardiovascular disease, such as strokes and heart attacks (see Sect. 5.2), which is why they should be used only for short periods and only in people with a healthy cardiovascular system. In some countries, coxibs are not approved, because of their associated ADRs.

What to Do if You Take Cortisone, Acetylsalicylic Acid, or Clopidogrel

Glucocorticoids ("cortisone" or, more precisely, cortisone derivatives; the prototype drug is prednisolone) have mainly anti-inflammatory effects and are therefore used in many autoimmune diseases (see Sect. 11.2). Glucocorticoids have many effects on inflammatory processes. One of their effects (as with NSAIDs) is inhibition of prostaglandin formation, which is why they can cause PUD. One can try to use more specific anti-inflammatory drugs or reduce the dose of the glucocorticoid. Additional administration of a PPI is possible.

A special situation occurs when a patient is treated with low-dose ASA or clopidogrel over a long period to prevent a heart attack or a stroke. Both drugs inhibit platelet aggregation in the blood (see Sect. 5.2). This mechanism prevents heart attacks and strokes but promotes development of PUD. However, long-term therapy with ASA or clopidogrel is necessary to prevent life-threatening cardiovascular events. Therefore, discontinuation of the drugs is not a viable alternative. It is therefore advisable to regularly check these patients for blood in their stools, using appropriate laboratory tests, or to measure hemoglobin in the blood to detect any (minor) bleeding. If indicated, an endoscopy should be carried out to detect an ulcer. Only if an ulcer is diagnosed is concomitant treatment with a PPI appropriate. Routine prescribing of a PPI during treatment with ASA or clopidogrel is problematic because PPIs can cause dangerous ADRs with long-term use (see Sect. 3.1).

3.3 Constipation and Diarrhea

Summary

The most common causes of constipation are a diet low in fiber, lack of exercise, inadequate fluid intake, potassium deficiency, and regular use of laxatives. Diabetes, hypothyroidism, multiple sclerosis, and depression can promote constipation. The key is to eliminate the causes and treat the underlying conditions. In the case of constipation caused by opioid analgesics, administration of macrogol, which enlarges and softens the intestinal contents, is essential. Viral infections are the most common cause of diarrhea. Certain drugs can cause diarrhea. This is especially true of antibiotics, which can damage the intestinal microbiome. The focuses of treatment are elimination of the causes of diarrhea and replacement of fluids. For symptomatic treatment, loperamide can be used in the short term.

Memo

- Constipation is prevented by a diet rich in fiber and potassium, sufficient fluid intake, and exercise.
- Regular use of laxatives promotes constipation.
- Without adequate fluid intake, intake of wheat bran and flaxseed can cause constipation.
- Use of diuretics, parasympatholytic drugs, aluminum-containing antacids. and opioid analgesics can cause constipation.
- Laxatives should be used only for short periods, except during treatment with opioid analgesics.
- In the event of diarrhea caused by a virus, the focus is on symptomatic treatment.
- Loperamide reduces stool frequency, metoclopramide alleviates nausea and vomiting, and butylscopolamine relieves intestinal cramps.
- Several drugs, including antibiotics and magnesium-containing antacids, can cause diarrhea.

How Does Constipation Occur?

Figure 3.3 shows how constipation and diarrhea occur and how they are treated. Table 3.3 summarizes the most important drugs used in treatment of constipation and diarrhea. It is a common misconception that you must have a bowel movement every day. We speak of constipation if bowel movements are less frequent than three times a week. Constipation becomes more frequent with age and reduced mobility. Women are more prone to constipation than men.

Lack of fluid intake, insufficient physical activity, and a diet low in fiber are common causes of constipation. They are easy to treat through lifestyle changes.

Chronic diseases such as diabetes (see Sect. 6.1), Parkinson disease (see Sect. 8.1), hypothyroidism (see Sect. 6.2), depression (see Sect. 9.2), colon cancer, or hemorrhoids can cause constipation. Constipation improves when the underlying condition is properly treated.

Why You Should Not Take Laxatives Regularly

If you suffer from constipation, taking one of the numerous available laxatives seems to be an easy solution to the problem. Many laxatives are herbal and thus supposedly "natural". The over-the-counter availability of laxatives suggests they are harmless. This assumption is supported by clever advertising, as many laxatives are promoted with an undefined promise of wellness or detoxification.

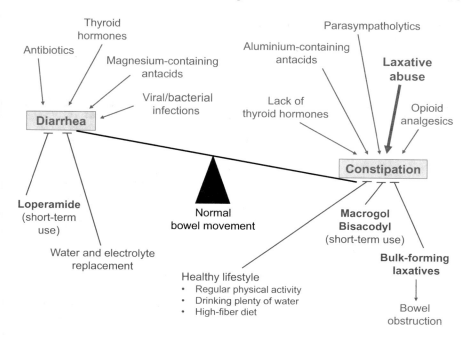

Fig. 3.3 Why do constipation and diarrhea occur, and how are they treated? Diarrhea and constipation can be viewed as a deviation from the balance (homeostasis) of intestinal function. With diarrhea, nausea and vomiting are often present as well. Metoclopramide (see Sect. 3.1) can be used to treat these symptoms. Parasympatholytics (the prototype drug is butylscopolamine) are suitable for treatment of intestinal cramps. For the sake of clarity, those aspects are not shown in this figure. Except for pain management with opioid analgesics (see Sects. 2.2 and 11.1), long-term treatment with laxatives must be avoided. Abuse of laxatives (often for many years) is the most important cause of chronic constipation. A healthy lifestyle is crucial in treatment of constipation

The danger of all laxatives is that they cause loss of water and potassium, which is an unavoidable part of their action. Potassium deficiency decreases bowel activity and thus can worsen constipation. As a result, regular use of laxatives can develop a vicious cycle between constipation and laxative use. Therefore, it is recommended to have your serum potassium concentration ("potassium level") determined by your doctor in the event of constipation.

The key to overcoming this vicious cycle is a diet rich in fiber (e.g., cereals, fruit, and vegetables), adequate intake of potassium (e.g., in orange juice, pistachios, soy, apricots, and wheat bran), and sufficient intake of fluid (e.g., 1.5–2 liters of mineral water per day). Adequate exercise (such as walking, running, and gym exercise) stimulates bowel movements as well.

Table 3.3 Overview of the most important drug classes used for treatment of constipation and diarrhea

Drug class	Prototype drug	Mechanisms of action	Indications	Important adverse drug reactions (ADRs) and interactions
Stimulatory laxatives	Bisacodyl	Absorption of water and salts in the intestine is inhibited; at the same time, excretion of water and salts is promoted	Short-term use for severe constipation (e.g., before surgery and in hemorrhoids)	Loss of water and salt, especially with long-term use (abuse); this can worsen constipation in a vicious cycle; intestinal cramps
Parasympatholytics	Butylscopolamine	Muscarinic receptor antagonism, relaxation of intestinal muscles, inhibition of intestinal activity	Analgesic effect in intestinal spasms; the muscle-relaxing effect can be used in uterine spasms (e.g., during menstruation)	Constipation and urinary retention with excessive use (antimuscarinic syndrome)
Opioid receptor agonists	Loperamide	Opioid receptor agonism acting only in the intestine (but not in the brain); slowing of bowel activity; thus, less urge to defecate and fewer bowel movements; loperamide does *not* have analgesic effects	Short-term treatment of (viral) diarrhea with frequent bowel movements; used when the underlying cause of diarrhea cannot be eliminated and water and salt replacement are not sufficient	To avoid constipation, use this therapy only until the first normally formed stools are produced; forbidden in infants and young children because respiratory arrest may occur; forbidden in cases of bloody diarrhea and fever because excretion of pathogens may be delayed

(continued)

Table 3.3 (continued)

Drug class	Prototype drug	Mechanisms of action	Indications	Important adverse drug reactions (ADRs) and interactions
Water-binding laxatives	Macrogol	Binding of water; improved bowel action by enlargement of intestinal contents; facilitated defecation by softening of intestinal contents	Short-term treatment of chronic constipation until lifestyle modification measures take effect; prevention of constipation during opioid analgesic therapy	Water and salt losses with long-term use; thus, aggravation of constipation; well tolerated; no flatulence and no intestinal cramps (in contrast to lactulose)
Water and salt replacement	WHO (World Health Organization) rehydration solution with water, glucose, and various salts	Replacement of water and salt lost from the body	Severe diarrhea with marked signs of dehydration and risk of water thrombosis (thickening of the blood)	Very well tolerated when used properly; risk of water retention in the body with excessive use

Use of metoclopramide (MCP) for treatment of nausea and vomiting is discussed in Sect. 3.1 and Table 1.1

ADR adverse drug reaction, *MCP* metoclopramide, *WHO* World Health Organization

Which Drugs Can Cause Constipation?

Constipation is caused by many drugs. A prominent example is constipation caused by opioid analgesics. As these drugs are often used for serious and life-threatening conditions such as cancer (see Sects. 2.2 and 11.1), constipation caused by opioid analgesics must be treated from the outset. Macrogol is the most suitable drug for this purpose.

Use of calcium channel blockers for treatment of high blood pressure (see Sect. 5.1), use of iron preparations for treatment of anemia, and use of PPIs and aluminum-containing antacids for self-treatment of GERD (see Sect. 3.1) are frequent causes of constipation. For a variety of diseases, parasympatholytics are used. These drugs block the activity of the parasympathetic system, which is responsible for normal digestive activity. As a result, intestinal activity is inhibited and constipation thus occurs. Drugs with a parasympatholytic effect include scopolamine (which is used for motion sickness), first-generation antihistamines (which are used for allergies; see Sect. 4.1), antidepressant nonselective monoamine reuptake inhibitors (NSMRIs; see Sect. 9.2), many antipsychotics (see Sect. 9.4), and biperiden, which is used to treat Parkinson disease (see Sect. 8.1).

Diuretics such as chlorthalidone (a weaker diuretic) and furosemide (a stronger diuretic), which are often used to treat high blood pressure and heart failure (see Sects. 5.1 and 5.3), can cause potassium deficiency and thus affect digestive activity. Therefore, they are often combined with potassium-sparing drugs such as angiotensin-converting enzyme (ACE) inhibitors or angiotensin receptor blockers (ARBs; see Sects. 5.1–5.3).

Which Laxative Should You Take?

Table 3.3 summarizes important drugs for treatment of constipation and diarrhea. With the exception of treatment of pain with opioid analgesics, laxatives should be used only for a short time and only for a good reason. For most patients, macrogol is the best laxative because it is slow acting, mild, and well tolerated. It absorbs water from the intestines like a sponge. This makes the intestinal contents softer and larger, which stimulates bowel movements. When using macrogol, it is essential to ensure adequate fluid intake.

Lactulose is often used. This is a sugar that cannot be broken down in the small intestine. Lactulose is broken down in the large intestine by bacteria. The resulting short-chain fatty acids stimulate intestinal activity. Lactulose is not as well tolerated as macrogol. Degradation of lactulose by intestinal bacteria can cause gas, bloating, flatulence, intestinal cramps, and nausea. These ADRs do not occur with macrogol.

Dietary fibers such as wheat bran and linseed are popular as well. If you take these, you must drink a lot of liquid, because otherwise the stools harden and causes painful bowel movements. Consuming extra wheat bran and flaxseed is unnecessary if you get enough fiber in your diet. A first step is to eat whole-grain bread.

Several laxatives irritate the intestinal mucosa. As a result, more water and salts are excreted into the intestine, and they are less absorbed from there into the body. Overall, these drugs are more aggressive than macrogol. They can cause significant water and salt loss, as well as intestinal cramping. Bisacodyl is the prototype of such a drug. When it is administered orally, the effect occurs after 6–8 hours; when it is administered as a suppository, it occurs within 1–3 hours.

What Causes Diarrhea?

Diarrhea is defined as more than three bowel movements a day, with unformed (liquid) stools and a stool weight exceeding 200 g per discharge. Diarrhea is often accompanied by strong intestinal cramps. The stools are often profusely splashed and have a foul odor, which reflects disturbance of the intestinal microbiome (see Sect. 11.3). Nausea and vomiting are common symptoms in diarrhea.

Approximately 75% of all diarrheal cases are caused by viruses. Viral diarrhea is common, especially in the summertime. This "summer flu" cannot be treated causally; only its prevailing symptoms can be treated.

In rarer cases, bacteria cause diarrhea. Usually, the symptoms are more severe than those of diarrhea caused by viruses. Fever, bloody stools, and a poor general condition are typical symptoms of bacterial diarrhea. In these cases, it is essential to consult a doctor.

Another common cause of diarrhea is hyperthyroidism or use of thyroid hormones (see Sect. 6.2). If a patient needs thyroid hormone (levothyroxine, T4) because of hypothyroidism, it is essential that T4 is taken with water at least half an hour before breakfast. Failure to do so may result in diarrhea (see Sect. 6.2).

Other causes of diarrhea are autoimmune diseases such as ulcerative colitis and Crohn disease. In these diseases, the focus is on treatment with drugs that suppress the excessive activity of the immune system. This therapy improves the diarrhea (see Sect. 11.2).

A common cause of diarrhea is treatment with antibiotics (see Sect. 11.3), which are used for diseases caused by bacteria (e.g., upper respiratory tract infections, pneumonia, or urinary tract infections). Antibiotics not only damage the disease-causing bacteria but also disturb the balance of the intestinal microbiome and thus often lead to diarrhea. Any antibiotic can cause diarrhea. In such a case, the doctor and patient must discuss whether a switch to another antibiotic must be made.

Short-term, high-dose use of laxatives, especially irritant laxatives, can cause diarrhea. Laxatives are often used (in combination with diuretics) to reduce body weight by models or athletes who are competing in weight classes. This abuse is dangerous and can lead to water and salt loss, which reduces physical performance. In addition, use of magnesium-containing antacids can cause diarrhea. These drugs are often used for self-medication of GERD (see Sect. 3.1).

How to Treat Diarrhea

Whenever possible, it is crucial to find the cause of the diarrhea and to eliminate it. Otherwise, the treatment is symptom oriented. It is most important to prevent severe water and salt losses, as these can lead to weakening of the body and thickening of the blood, with a risk of thrombosis. Accordingly, water and salts must be supplied to the body. Supply of water alone is not sufficient.

An old and effective remedy for mild diarrhea is to drink cola with salt sticks. This "treatment" is based on the fact that glucose (the sugar component in cola), salt from the salt sticks, and water are absorbed from the intestine through a common pathway (a pump; see Sect. 1.4). It is possible to make a drinking solution from salt and sugar mixtures packed in sachets. These sachets are available in a wide variety of flavors. The reconstituted drinking solution is called WHO (World Health Organization) rehydration solution. In case of severe diarrhea, up to 3 liters of fluid must be consumed per day. If a patient has a poor physical status, fluid and salt are replaced by intravenous infusion.

Opioid analgesics have a constipating effect. Loperamide is used for symptomatic treatment of diarrhea. It acts through the same receptors as opioid analgesics (so it is an opioid receptor agonist). However, unlike opioid analgesics (see Sect. 2.2), loperamide has no effect in the brain. Therefore, loperamide does not relieve pain, does not make you tired, and does not suppress your breathing. It inhibits bowel activity and thus reduces the urge to have a bowel movement and the frequency of bowel movements. Loperamide can be used for short-term treatment of mild diarrhea (especially of viral origin).

Loperamide should not be used in severe diarrhea with fever and blood in the stools. Such diarrhea could be caused by bacteria. Suppression of diarrhea delays elimination of pathogens and thus prolongs the course of the disease. Loperamide should not be used in infants and young children. In this age group, the drug can easily enter the brain and cause respiratory arrest (see Sect. 1.5). In schoolchildren, loperamide is dosed according to body weight. Loperamide should be used only for short periods. Its misuse leads to constipation.

Diarrhea is often accompanied by severe intestinal cramps, which can be treated with butylscopolamine, a parasympatholytic drug (muscarinic receptor antagonist). Metoclopramide (MCP) can be used for nausea and vomiting associated with viral diarrhea. These drugs are discussed in Sect. 3.1. Like loperamide and butylscopolamine, metoclopramide should be used only for short periods. Metoclopramide is not allowed in infants and young children, because it can enter the brain and cause harmless but awkward-looking movement disorders (dyskinesias; see Sects. 1.5 and 3.1).

4

Drugs for Respiratory Diseases

Abstract Allergies are caused by malfunction of the immune system. The decisive factor in the treatment of allergies is (if possible) avoidance of the causative allergen. Wheals, conjunctivitis, and rhinitis are treated with antihistamines. Short- and long-acting beta sympathomimetics, inhaled corticosteroids, and leukotriene receptor antagonists are the main drugs used for treatment of asthma. Anaphylactic shock is a life-threatening form of allergy. The most important measure in anaphylactic shock is an injection of epinephrine (adrenaline). Self-therapy with epinephrine can be lifesaving. In chronic obstructive pulmonary disease, irreversible dilation of the alveoli occurs, usually because of decades of tobacco consumption. Accordingly, giving up tobacco products is the most effective form of treatment for chronic obstructive pulmonary disease, a condition that cannot be cured, only treated symptomatically. Chronic obstructive pulmonary disease is treated with long-acting beta sympathomimetics and long-acting antimuscarinics. Use of inhaled corticosteroids in chronic obstructive pulmonary disease is dangerous because they increase the risk of pneumonia.

4.1   Allergies and Asthma

Summary

Allergies are caused by malfunction of the immune system. Harmless components of the environment lead to increased formation of immunoglobulin E (IgE). It activates mast cells, which release mediators of inflammation. These include histamine and leukotrienes, which in turn cause allergic symptoms. The spectrum ranges from wheals, conjunctivitis, and rhinitis to asthma attacks and potentially fatal anaphylactic (allergic) shock. The most important action (if possible) is to avoid allergens. Wheals, conjunctivitis, and rhinitis are treated with antihistamines. Asthma is treated with short-acting beta sympathomimetics (SABAs), long-acting beta sympathomimetics (LABAs), inhaled glucocorticoids (ICSs), and leukotriene receptor antagonists (LTRAs). In treatment of anaphylactic shock, epinephrine (EPI, adrenaline) is lifesaving.

Memo

- Wheals, conjunctivitis, and rhinitis are treated with antihistamines.
- First-generation antihistamines enter the brain and cause fatigue.
- Second-generation antihistamines pose a lower risk of fatigue.
- Antihistamines are not effective in asthma and insufficient in anaphylactic shock.
- In asthma, SABAs are used first, followed by ICSs, which are often given in combination with LABAs.
- For severe asthma, LTRAs are added.
- Epinephrine (adrenaline) is the key drug in anaphylactic shock, both in treatment by a doctor and in self-therapy.

How Do Allergies and Asthma Develop?

Allergies are divided into four classes (types I–IV). Here, only type I allergy is discussed. It is the most common form of allergy. It is not yet known why some people develop allergies and others do not. Allergens are substances that can trigger allergic reactions. Figure 4.1 shows the development of type I allergies and drug therapy. Allergens can include flower pollen, food components, and mite excrement. Certain drugs can trigger allergies. Particularly dangerous, but often underestimated, is use of sulfonamides (which are combined with trimethoprim in the antibiotic cotrimoxazole) for urinary tract infections (see Sect. 11.3).

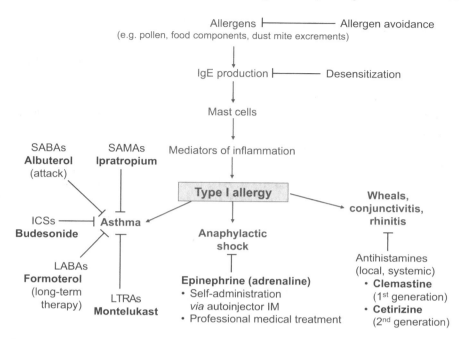

Fig. 4.1 How do allergies and asthma develop, and how are they treated? Treatment of asthma, on the one hand, and treatment of wheals, conjunctivitis, and rhinitis, on the other hand, differ because different mediators of inflammation (see Sect. 1.5) are involved. Antihistamines are ineffective in treatment of asthma and are insufficient in treatment of anaphylactic (allergic) shock. In this case, treatment with epinephrine (adrenaline) is lifesaving. You can administer epinephrine yourself. You will be trained by your doctor and receive an epinephrine auto-injector (or two). In this way, you can save your life until an emergency doctor takes over further treatment. The importance of glucocorticoids ("cortisone") in emergency treatment of anaphylactic shock is over-rated. Unlike epinephrine, they take effect not within seconds but only after several hours. However, seconds do matter. Another common mistake is overdosing on antihistamines. This leads to an antimuscarinic syndrome

Because of a malfunction in the immune system, antibodies (immuno-globulins) from the IgE class are formed in the body and act against the aller-gens. Detection of an increased IgE concentration in the blood is an indication of a predisposition to allergic reactions. When IgE antibodies bind their aller-gen (antigen), activation of mast cells takes place. Mast cells are filled with vesicles that contain various mediators of inflammation, including histamine and leukotrienes. Mast cells are found mainly in the skin, eyes, respiratory system, and gastrointestinal tract. Their normal role is to monitor the body against cancer cells, bacteria, and parasites (see Sects. 11.1 and 11.3). Mast cells therefore have a useful function. However, in the context of allergic reac-tions, they are inappropriately activated.

From Harmless to Life Threatening

Symptoms differ depending on the region of the body in which the mast cells are activated by allergens. If the conjunctiva of the eyes is affected, conjunctivitis develops (allergic conjunctivitis). If the mucous membrane of the nose is affected, hay fever develops (allergic rhinitis). If the mast cells in the skin are activated, wheals form (urticaria). These forms of allergy are characterized by redness, edema, and itching.

If the mast cells in the airways—especially those the small bronchi (bronchioles)—are activated, they contract. As a result, shortness of breath occurs, particularly during exhalation (asthma). If mast cells are activated throughout the body, vasodilation and a drop in blood pressure develop, with reduced blood flow to the organs. This life-threatening condition is called anaphylactic (allergic) shock.

Type I allergies can therefore present themselves in different ways, from harmless to life threatening. A localized allergic reaction can spread and become life threatening. The course is unpredictable.

General Therapy

An important therapeutic strategy for type I allergies is to avoid the triggering allergen. This is often easier said than done, because provocation tests do not always a succeed in finding the trigger or because it is impossible to avoid it in daily life.

A popular strategy for treating allergies is to desensitize the body. After the doctor has identified the allergen, increasing doses of the allergen are administered to the patient in the skin (intradermally) at regular intervals and over a longer period. The idea behind this therapy is that the body produces more "good" antibodies of the immunoglobulin G (IgG) class, which intercept the allergen and thus prevent mast cell activation by the "bad" IgE.

However, desensitization therapy is problematic because, after each allergen administration, the patient must remain in the doctor's office for at least 30–45 minutes to ensure that no anaphylactic shock develops. Because of the effort involved in desensitization, adherence to therapy is low and its success is uncertain.

Therefore, drug treatment of allergies is important. Although the various forms of type I allergy have a common mechanism, the treatments used for individual manifestations differ significantly from each other. Table 4.1 summarizes important drugs used in treatment of type I allergy.

Table 4.1 Overview of the most important drug classes used for treatment of type I allergies

Drug class	Prototype drug	Mechanisms of action	Indications	Important adverse drug reactions (ADRs) and interactions
First-generation antihistamines	Clemastine	Block the effects of histamine released from mast cells; H₁ receptor antagonism; block the effects of histamine in the brain; rapid onset of action; well tolerated if used properly	Oral or intravenous administration in severe allergic reactions manifesting as wheals, conjunctivitis, or rhinitis; local application on the skin to relieve small wheals and itching; motion sickness; difficulties in falling asleep; no effect in asthma	Fatigue; traffic safety and ability to operate machinery are impaired; increased drowsiness with consumption of alcohol and other drugs with effects on the brain, especially benzodiazepines, Z-drugs, and antiepileptic drugs; in long-term use, weight gain due to increased appetite
Second-generation antihistamines	Cetirizine	Block the effects of histamine released from mast cells; H₁ receptor antagonism; little effect in the brain; rapid onset of action	Oral administration in allergic reactions manifesting as wheals, conjunctivitis, or rhinitis; local application as eye drops or nasal spray; only a slight effect on the brain; therefore, not to be used for difficulty falling asleep or for motion sickness; no effect in asthma	Overall good tolerability; temporary bitter taste or burning sensation after local application; fatigue may occur in sensitive individuals, especially at higher doses

(continued)

Table 4.1 (continued)

Drug class	Prototype drug	Mechanisms of action	Indications	Important adverse drug reactions (ADRs) and interactions
Short-acting muscarinic antagonists (SAMAs)	**Ipratropium**	Block the effects of acetylcholine on the bronchi; muscarinic receptor antagonism (parasympatholytic); dilation of airways; relievers	Inhalation during a severe asthma attack	Overall good tolerability; dry mouth if inhaled incorrectly
Short-acting beta agonists (SABAs, short-acting beta sympathomimetics)	**Albuterol**	Mimic the effects of epinephrine on the bronchi; beta-2 receptor agonism; dilate airways; rapid onset but short duration of action; relievers	Inhalation during an acute asthma attack; on-demand medication	Good tolerability when used correctly; bitter taste with incorrect inhalation technique; palpitations with overdose; risk of angina pectoris attacks in patients with coronary heart disease (CHD); loss of effect after too frequent use
Long-acting beta agonists (LABAs, long-acting beta sympathomimetics)	**Formoterol**	Mimic the effects of epinephrine on the bronchi; beta-2 receptor agonism; dilate airways; slow onset but long duration of action; controllers	Long-term treatment of asthma; prevention of asthma attacks; regular inhalation	Tremors, headaches, restlessness, palpitations, elevation of blood glucose, especially with high doses; to avoid ADRs, combination with an inhaled corticosteroid (ICS) is recommended

Corticosteroids (glucocorticoids), inhaled corticosteroids (ICSs)	Budesonide	Inhibit the inflammatory response in asthma through several mechanisms and enhance the effect of SABAs and LABAs; contrary to widespread belief, they have no acute effect, only a prophylactic effect; controllers	Basic therapy for asthma; because it is applied as an inhaled spray, hardly any effects of the "cortisone" are to be expected in the body; locally applied corticosteroids for the conjunctiva and nose are available	Overall good tolerability if used correctly; *no risk of Cushing syndrome*, as budesonide is broken down rapidly in the liver; hoarseness and oral thrush (candidiasis) with incorrect application; hence, rinse the mouth after each application
Catecholamines	Epinephrine (EPI, adrenaline)	Dilation of airways; increases in cardiac output and organ blood flow; reduction of swelling in the face and neck area; relief from wheals; rapid onset of action	Anaphylactic shock; intravenous administration by an emergency doctor; epinephrine auto-injector for (intramuscular) self-injection by patients with known allergies	Very good tolerability if used and dosed correctly, as the effect is limited in time; in patients with high blood pressure, risk of further increase in blood pressure; in patients with CHD, risk of angina pectoris and myocardial infarction; however, these ADRs can be controlled by an emergency doctor and take a back seat to the life-threatening situation

(continued)

Table 4.1 (continued)

Drug class	Prototype drug	Mechanisms of action	Indications	Important adverse drug reactions (ADRs) and interactions
Leukotriene receptor antagonists (LTRAs)	**Montelukast**	Inhibit the effects of leukotrienes on the bronchi, thereby dilating airways and reducing inflammation; delayed onset of effect; hence, suited to prophylactic treatment; controllers	Long-term treatment of asthma if SABA, LABA, and ICS therapies are not sufficient	Gastric/intestinal complaints, headaches

Drug-specific word stems are shown in bold text. If you have ever experienced anaphylactic shock, ask your doctor to prescribe at least two epinephrine auto-injectors (in case one doesn't work) and carry them with you. Instruct your family members and friends how to use an epinephrine auto-injector when in doubt. These simple measures can save your life. Do not waste time taking antihistamines in anaphylactic shock; they do *not* work for asthma. Theophylline is described in Sect. 4.2

ADR adverse drug reaction, *CHD* coronary heart disease, *ICS* inhaled corticosteroid, *LABA* long-acting beta agonist, *LTRA* leukotriene receptor antagonist, *SABA* short-acting beta agonist, *SAMA* short-acting muscarinic antagonist

Drugs for Wheals, Conjunctivitis, and Rhinitis

Wheals, conjunctivitis, and rhinitis are unpleasant but not life-threatening manifestations of type I allergy. In these manifestations, itching, redness, and edema are the main symptoms. Itching becomes more severe if you. Generalized wheals are an alarm sign. They can be an indication that the allergic reaction is spreading throughout the body.

In the aforementioned manifestations of allergy, histamine is the most important mediator of inflammation. It binds to histamine H_1 receptors, thereby triggering blood vessel dilation, redness, edema, and itching. Accordingly, the most important and successful therapy is to antagonize (block) the effects of histamine at these receptors. Antihistamines bind to H_1 receptors in competition with histamine, which can now no longer act (see Sect. 1.4).

Depending on whether symptoms are localized or generalized, either local therapy (with eye drops, nasal spray, or skin gel) or systemic therapy (with tablets) must be used. A major advantage of antihistamines is that they act within a few minutes. It is therefore possible, at the onset of allergy symptoms, to use the drug for a short time (on demand) until the symptoms stop. In most cases, this strategy is sufficient. In the case of seasonal allergy (e.g., to certain plant pollens), therapy with antihistamines can be carried out during the corresponding season to prevent the onset of allergy symptoms.

A variety of antihistamines are available on the drug market. Some antihistamines do not require a prescription. A distinction is made between first- and second-generation antihistamines. First-generation drugs (the prototype drugs are clemastine and diphenhydramine) inhibit not just the effects of histamine on the allergic reaction but also those in the brain. In the brain, histamine promotes attention, inhibits appetite, and triggers motion sickness. Accordingly, by blocking the effects of histamine in the brain, first-generation antihistamines cause fatigue and increased appetite, and they suppress symptoms of motion sickness. Antihistamines of the second generation reach the brain to a much lesser extent than those of the first generation, and so they cause less fatigue.

If a patient takes an oral first-generation antihistamine because of an allergic reaction, the symptoms of wheals, conjunctivitis, and rhinitis are reduced, but the patient becomes tired. This sleep-inducing effect of first-generation antihistamines can be used in the case of sleep disorders but does significantly impair the ability to drive. Additional consumption of alcoholic beverages or use of benzodiazepines or Z-drugs exacerbates the problem (see Sect. 8.2). It is therefore essential that car drivers avoid oral administration of first-generation antihistamines.

The risks of fatigue and impaired driving are lower with second-generation antihistamines (the prototype drugs are cetirizine and fexofenadine). Some people get tired after taking second-generation antihistamines. In this case, it is recommended to switch to another second-generation antihistamine or try a lower dose.

It is a common mistake to use excessive doses of antihistamines to treat allergic symptoms. This is because other mediators of inflammation besides histamine play a role in allergy, and in higher doses, antihistamines block muscarinic receptors (i.e., they act as parasympatholytics [antimuscarinics]). This can lead to adverse drug reactions (ADRs) such as a dry mouth; hot, dry skin; palpitations; constipation; urinary retention; and blurred vision. These symptoms are grouped under the term "antimuscarinic syndrome" (or "anticholinergic syndrome").

A wide range of second-generation antihistamines are available for use in the eyes, for use in the nose, and for oral administration. You should discuss the best form of application with your doctor and pharmacist. When antihistamines are applied locally to a small area, systemic ADRs hardly occur; they are to be expected only with oral therapy. Antihistamines are safe and effective if these rules for their use are observed.

Asthma Therapy

While histamine plays a central role in development of wheals, conjunctivitis, and rhinitis, it is not involved in asthma. Accordingly, antihistamines are ineffective in asthma.

The leading symptom of asthma is shortness of breath, especially during exhalation. In asthma, because of mast cell activation, narrowing of the airways and inflammation develop, which lead to thickening of the bronchial mucosa. Asthma is reversible. Drug therapy for asthma depends on its severity.

A peak flowmeter is an easy-to-use device to check the severity of your asthma on your own. It measures the maximum liters of air you can exhale per second. The peak expiratory flow (PEF) values depend on your age and sex, and can be checked against reference tables. In intermittent asthma, PEF values are reduced by up to 20% and no more than one asthma attack per week occurs. In mild asthma, the attack frequency increases to up to one attack per day. Moderate asthma, with PEF values reduced by 20–40%, is accompanied by daily attacks. In severe asthma, PEF values are reduced by more than 40%

and asthma attacks occur several times per day. The most severe life-threatening form of asthma is status asthmaticus. It must be treated as an emergency.

The goals of asthma treatment are freedom from attacks, normal lung function, and a good quality of life. These goals can be achieved with stage-appropriate drug therapy. A distinction is made between relievers, which improve acute asthma symptoms, and controllers, which reduce the frequency of attacks and inflammation in the bronchi in the long term. Short-acting beta sympathomimetics (short-acting beta receptor agonists, SABAs) and antimuscarinics (short-acting muscarinic receptor antagonists, SAMAs) are relievers. Inhaled corticosteroids (ICSs, glucocorticoids), long-acting beta sympathomimetics (long-acting beta receptor agonists, LABAs), and leukotriene receptor antagonists (LTRAs) are controllers.

Short-Acting and Long-Acting Beta Receptor Agonists

Initially, SABAs (the prototype drugs are albuterol and fenoterol) are used on demand for mild asthma. Correct intake of each drug, coordinated with inhalation, is crucial. Your doctor and pharmacist will show you the correct inhalation technique. A bitter taste after inhalation points to incorrect inhalation, which is due to the drug remaining in the mouth.

A common problem with the use of SABAs is impatience on the part of the patient. The patient has shortness of breath and wants to have fast relief. However, before the drug reaches the site of action (the smooth muscle cells in the bronchi), approximately 3–4 minutes pass. This interval cannot be shortened. It is a mistake, however, if you immediately take another puff of the inhalation spray because of the initial lack of effect of the SABA. You will experience heart palpitations when you start to breathe better again. This is because the higher doses of SABA activate the corresponding receptors for epinephrine (adrenaline) in the heart. The resulting increase in the heart rate is unfavorable in patients with heart disease and high blood pressure (see Sects. 5.1 and 5.2).

Another risk arises if a patient must inhale a SABA more frequently than twice a day to be symptom-free. In addition to the effect of an ADR on the heart, this can lead to a reduction of the drug's effect on the airways. This is due to a protective mechanism of the body against overactivation: the corresponding receptors in the airways disappear when overstimulated. The only way to restore sensitivity to SABAs is to discontinue use of the drug. During this period, the patient will feel worse at first.

LABAs have a significantly longer effect than SABAs. However, treatment with a LABA alone results in the same problems as those seen with a SABA. Therefore, LABAs are used in combination with ICSs in asthma.

Cortisone

Because of the disadvantages of treatment with a SABA or LABA alone, asthma patients should inhale an ICS (the prototype drug is budesonide) at an early stage. Many patients associate "steroids" or "cortisone" with severe ADRs (see Sect. 11.2). This leads to undertreatment and worsening of their asthma.

Modern ICSs are effective anti-inflammatory drugs and enhance the dilating effect of SABAs and LABAs on the bronchi. Since ICSs are applied by inhalation and are broken down rapidly in the body, the effects of ICSs are limited to the airways.

It is often thought that the main problem with asthma is bronchoconstriction. However, inflammation, which is relieved by ICSs, is similarly problematic. In addition, ICSs increase the number of receptors for SABAs and LABAs on the smooth muscle cells of the bronchi, thereby enhancing the effects of beta sympathomimetics.

As with SABAs and LABAs, use of a proper inhalation technique is important with ICSs. As they affect the immune system, susceptibility to infections may be increased. Of particular importance is oral candidiasis (see Sect. 11.3), caused by the yeast *Candida albicans*, which is part of the normal microbiome. When ICSs are present in higher concentrations, yeast can dominate the microbiome. Candidiasis can be recognized by whitish coatings on reddened mucosa, which bleeds easily. Infection can be prevented by use of a proper inhalation technique. It is recommended to rinse the mouth after each inhalation of ICS to remove any drug left behind. Another ADR caused by ICSs is hoarseness, which may necessitate a dose reduction.

More Options

If asthma is not adequately controlled by SABA + LABA + ICS, leukotriene receptor antagonists (LTRAs) can be given additionally. These drugs prevent inflammation and constriction of the bronchi caused by leukotrienes.

In asthma, the SAMA ipratropium can be used as a further reliever. For severe cases, the reliever theophylline is available. However, it acts not only in the airways but everywhere in the body; thus, severe ADRs such as nausea, vomiting, diarrhea, palpitations, tremors, and agitation can occur (see Sect. 4.2).

In most cases, asthma can be controlled by a combination of SABA + LABA + ICS + LTRA. However, a few patients do not respond to this standard therapy. For them, special (and expensive) drugs can be used. Omalizumab is an antibody that binds to IgE and prevents mast cell activation. The antibody mepolizumab reduces inflammation by binding to the mediator of inflammation interleukin-5 (IL-5).

Aspirin-Induced Asthma

At this point, aspirin-induced asthma must be mentioned. Approximately 15% of all asthma patients have hypersensitivity to nonsteroidal anti-inflammatory drugs (NSAIDs). These drugs inhibit formation of prostaglandins and thus reduce pain caused by inflammation (see Sect. 2.1). In return, however, the body produces more leukotrienes, which constrict the airways and worsen asthma. However, the term "aspirin-induced asthma" is misleading because it is not only acetylsalicylic acid (ASA) that causes this asthma; all other NSAIDs (such as ibuprofen) do too. Paracetamol and metamizole do not cause aspirin-induced asthma (see Sect. 2.1).

Anaphylactic Shock

Anaphylactic (allergic) shock is the most severe, life-threatening form of type I allergy. It can develop from a harmless allergic reaction. Warning symptoms for development of anaphylactic shock are wheals that spread rapidly over the whole body and itch intensely, swelling in the face and neck, and shortness of breath. As a result, organs are deprived of oxygen. Furthermore, gastrointestinal symptoms such as nausea, vomiting, and diarrhea may occur. Massive dilation of blood vessels with a resulting drop in blood pressure and reduced supply of oxygen and nutrients to organs can develop. Initially, the heart attempts to improve the reduced blood supply by increasing its output (this is recognizable by palpitations), but, ultimately, this no longer helps (the heart itself suffers from lack of nutrients and oxygen), and death ensues.

Treatment of Anaphylactic Shock

In allergic shock, treatment is needed as soon as possible. The patient must immediately call an emergency doctor or be taken to an emergency room. The most important and lifesaving measure in anaphylactic shock is intravenous administration of epinephrine (adrenaline). The doctor can dose it precisely in terms of its effect, and epinephrine acts in the body within seconds.

Epinephrine is often referred to as a "stress hormone". This bad reputation led to epinephrine being used too rarely in anaphylactic shock, resulting in avoidable deaths. Epinephrine is a life saver in anaphylactic shock. It reduces swelling in the head and neck, and it dilates the airways. This facilitates breathing and thus oxygenation of the body. Finally, epinephrine promotes heart function, facilitating distribution of oxygen throughout the body. Epinephrine thus combines three lifesaving effects in a single drug.

In the meantime, the attitude toward epinephrine has changed. Patients who have had anaphylactic shock are now prescribed an epinephrine auto-injector (or better still, two of them in case one fails or is used incorrectly) so they can inject themselves with the lifesaving epinephrine at the first sign of anaphylaxis.

Self-application of an epinephrine auto-injector must be explained by a doctor or pharmacist. The principle is that epinephrine is injected into a thigh muscle, using a syringe, with a self-release mechanism, that works even through clothing. An intramuscular injection is not as rapid and effective as an intravenous injection, but the epinephrine auto-injector gains valuable time until an emergency doctor arrives or the patient reaches an emergency room.

In the case of children who have had anaphylactic shock, parents and teachers must be instructed how to use an epinephrine auto-injector correctly. Accidental injection of the auto-injector contents into the user's finger does not lead to any long-term negative consequences. In the past, medical education recommended use of (high-dose) antihistamines and high-dose "cortisone" for treatment of anaphylactic shock, driven by the fear that use of epinephrine would be "stressful" for the patient. This practice resulted in deaths of patients from anaphylactic shock, which could have been prevented.

It must be emphasized, once again, that antihistamines *do not* act against bronchial constriction, *do not* act against facial and throat swelling, and *do not* act against cardiovascular symptoms; they act only against hives and itching. Contrary to popular belief, a higher antihistamine dose does not produce a better therapeutic effect; it only causes an antimuscarinic syndrome. Additionally administered H_2-receptor blockers for "stress ulcer prophylaxis" are not effective either.

Glucocorticoids are used in high doses with the idea that they will seal leaky blood vessels and prevent recurrence of anaphylaxis symptoms. The disadvantage of glucocorticoids is that the onset of action occurs within hours, although immediate action is required. Therefore, in an acute emergency, the focus of the patient and the doctor must be on intravenous or intramuscular administration of epinephrine.

4.2   Chronic Obstructive Pulmonary Disease

Summary

In chronic obstructive pulmonary disease (COPD), irreversible dilation of alveoli with narrowing of airways develops, usually because of tobacco use. The result is increasingly severe shortness of breath. COPD is incurable and can be treated only symptomatically. Initially, long-acting beta sympathomimetics (LABAs) and long-acting antimuscarinics (LAMAs) are used. Later, other bronchodilators such as the phosphodiesterase (PDE) inhibitors theophylline or roflumilast are applied. Glucocorticoids should be used cautiously because pneumonia can develop. At the final stage of COPD, pure oxygen is inhaled.

Memo

- The best prophylaxis and therapy for COPD is to refrain from using tobacco.
- The lung changes in COPD are irreversible.
- COPD is treated with inhaled LABAs and LAMAs.
- LABAs and LAMAs are effective and well tolerated.
- At the later stages of COPD, PDE inhibitors are used.
- Use of glucocorticoids is dangerous in COPD. Pneumonia can occur.
- At the late stages of COPD, pure oxygen must be inhaled.

How Does Chronic Obstructive Pulmonary Disease Develop?

In COPD, narrowing of small airways develops, resulting in impaired exhalation. In contrast to asthma, the lung changes in COPD are irreversible. The symptoms of COPD are shortness of breath, coughing, and sputum. Figure 4.2 shows how COPD develops and how it is treated.

The most important cause of COPD is long-term use of tobacco products. Tobacco contains many toxic substances that lead to chronic inflammation of small airways (bronchioles) and alveoli. The reduced number of alveoli makes oxygen uptake difficult, resulting in shortness of breath and a decline in physical capacity. The inflamed bronchioles collapse, especially during exhalation.

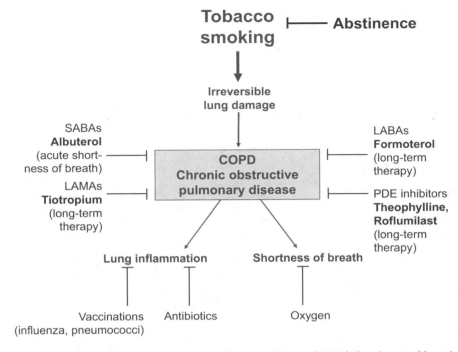

Fig. 4.2 How does chronic obstructive pulmonary disease (COPD) develop, and how is it treated? Treatment of COPD is symptomatic. A distinction is made between treatments for acute shortness of breath (short-acting beta agonists [SABAs] and oxygen) and long-term therapy (long-acting muscarinic antagonists [LAMAs], long-acting beta agonists [LABAs], and phosphodiesterase [PDE] inhibitors). Unlike asthma, COPD is not curable and, in most cases, leads to death. Only in a few cases is lung transplantation possible. The most important cause of COPD is tobacco smoke. Accordingly, abstaining from use of tobacco is the most effective treatment for COPD. Because of increased susceptibility to infection, glucocorticoids ("cortisone") should be avoided in COPD, if possible

This leads to air congestion in the lungs and further increases the damage. Eventually, emphysema develops. While asthma primarily affects young people, COPD is a disease of older people, usually manifesting after the age of 50 years. Accordingly, many COPD patients have cardiovascular disease (see Sects. 5.1–5.3), which complicates COPD treatment.

COPD is divided into four stages. The most important parameter is the forced expiratory volume in 1 second (FEV1). At stage 1 (mild COPD), the FEV1 is above 80% of normal and symptoms are mild. At stage 2 (moderate COPD), the FEV1 is reduced to 50–80% and symptoms become more evident. At stage 3 (severe COPD), the FEV1 is between 30% and 50%, with marked symptoms. At stage 4 (very severe COPD), the FEV1 is below 30% and breathlessness at rest is evident.

Short-Acting Beta Agonists and Long-Acting Muscarinic Antagonists

Table 4.2 provides an overview of the most important drugs for treatment of COPD. Since COPD cannot be cured, the aims are to alleviate symptoms and to improve physical performance. The key to success is abstinence from use of tobacco products. Influenza (flu) and pneumococcal vaccinations can mitigate the consequences of pneumonia in COPD.

Table 4.2 Overview of the most important drug classes used for treatment of chronic obstructive pulmonary disease (COPD)

Drug class	Prototype drug	Mechanisms of action	Indications	Important adverse drug reactions (ADRs) and interactions
Long-acting muscarinic antagonists (LAMAs)	Tio**tropium**	Muscarinic receptor antagonism (parasympatholytic) and dilation of airways	Inhalation in COPD; long-term use	Overall good tolerability; especially dry mouth in the event of incorrect inhalation
Phosphodiesterase (PDE) inhibitors	Theophylline	Dilation of airways and inhibition of inflammation; theophylline acts on all organs	Oral administration in severe forms of COPD; therapeutic drug monitoring (TDM) is required because of ADRs	Heart racing, heart palpitations, gastroesophageal reflux disease (GERD), diarrhea, nausea, vomiting, agitation, restlessness, tremors, seizures
Phosphodiesterase-4 (PDE4) inhibitors	Roflumi**last**	Dilation of airways and inhibition of inflammation; roflumilast acts more selectively on airways than theophylline	Oral administration in severe forms of COPD; more tolerable than theophylline	Nausea, vomiting, diarrhea, loss of appetite, sleep disorders, restlessness, tremors

Drug-specific word stems are shown in bold text. Short- and long-acting beta agonists (SABAs and LABAs) are discussed in Sect. 4.1. Unlike asthma, COPD is irreversible and cannot be cured. The drugs mentioned here have only symptomatic effects. You should therefore refrain from smoking tobacco products!

ADR adverse drug reaction, *COPD* chronic obstructive pulmonary disease, *GERD* gastroesophageal reflux disease, *LABA* long-acting beta agonist, *LAMA* long-acting muscarinic antagonist, *PDE* phosphodiesterase, *PDE4* phosphodiesterase-4, *SABA* short-acting beta agonist, *TDM* therapeutic drug monitoring

At stage 1, short-acting beta sympathomimetics (SABAs; the prototype drug is albuterol) are used as needed. These drugs are inhaled and lead to dilation of small airways. This facilitates exhalation. These drugs are discussed in Sect. 4.1.

At stage 2, long-acting muscarinic receptor antagonists (LAMAs, antimuscarinic agents, parasympatholytics) are given for long-term therapy (the prototype drug is tiotropium). These drugs are inhaled once daily. LAMAs cause airway dilation. Unlike SABAs, they are not suitable as an on-demand medication for acute symptom exacerbation. The advantages of LAMAs are that they are long acting and cause few ADRs when used correctly. The most unpleasant ADR is a dry mouth because tiotropium inhibits salivation. This ADR can be controlled by use of a good inhalation technique and rinsing of the mouth after inhalation.

Long-Acting Beta Agonists and Phosphodiesterase Inhibitors

If LAMAs are insufficient, long-acting beta sympathomimetics (LABAs) are added to the patient's treatment. The disadvantage of these drugs is that they can lose their effect when used long term. LABAs are discussed in detail in Sect. 4.1. For convenience, combinations of LABAs + LAMAs can be used.

Unfortunately, LABAs and LAMAs are often not sufficient to control symptoms. In these cases, other drug classes must be used. These include the phosphodiesterase (PDE) inhibitors theophylline and roflumilast. They inhibit breakdown of a second messenger called cyclic adenosine monophosphate (cAMP). PDE inhibitors have bronchodilatory and anti-inflammatory effects. Theophylline is a well-established drug for treatment of COPD; it works well but causes many ADRs. This is because it interferes with processes that occur in every cell in the body, not just in the airways and lungs. Thus, theophylline causes diarrhea, nausea and vomiting in the gastrointestinal tract, palpitations, and arrhythmias in the heart, as well as brain symptoms such as agitation, confusion, and seizures.

Because of the unfavorable ratio between desired effects and ADRs, theophylline must be dosed precisely to achieve an optimum effect for each patient. Regular determination of the drug concentration in the blood (therapeutic drug monitoring [TDM]) helps in this respect (see Sect. 1.5). Treatment with theophylline is complicated by the fact that it is broken down in the liver, which can lead to many interactions with other drugs. Use of theophylline is limited by ADRs.

COPD is often accompanied by coronary heart disease (CHD), which is also caused by (or at least aggravated by) use of tobacco products. The resulting need for treatment with many drugs (polypharmacy) increases the risk of interactions, particularly with theophylline.

Because of the disadvantages of theophylline, new drugs have been developed. One such new drug is roflumilast. Its mechanism of action and its effect are like those of theophylline. However, it acts more specifically on the respiratory tract and is therefore better tolerated.

Oxygen and Lung Transplantation

At the final stage of COPD, the number of alveoli for gas exchange has become so small that only administration of oxygen helps. However, constant dependence on an oxygen cylinder further restricts the mobility of patients.

Lung transplantation can be carried out in COPD, but donor organs are scarce. In addition, the heart is often so severely damaged that transplantation is not an option. After transplantation, immunosuppressive drugs must be taken to prevent rejection of the donor organ. Unfortunately, these drugs (the prototype drug is ciclosporin) increase susceptibility to infections (see Sects. 11.2 and 11.3). Another obstacle to transplantation is nicotine addiction. The best prevention and treatment for COPD is avoidance of tobacco products.

Caution with Cortisone

In COPD, inhaled glucocorticoids (corticosteroids, ICSs) must be used cautiously. These drugs weaken the body's defenses against infections, and pneumonia (bronchopneumonia) can develop. This can be severe in COPD and must be treated with an appropriate antibiotic. Whenever possible, antibiotics should be used in patients with COPD only after the pathogen has been identified and proven to be sensitive to the antibiotic (see Sect. 11.3). Macrolide antibiotics are frequently used for bronchopneumonia in COPD (Fig. 4.2 and Table 2.2).

5

Drugs for Cardiovascular Diseases

Abstract High blood pressure is often initially asymptomatic but must be treated right from the beginning. Otherwise, secondary diseases such as heart attack, stroke, heart failure, and arrhythmia may develop. In most patients, high blood pressure can be reduced with use of a drug in class A (inhibitors of the renin–angiotensin–aldosterone system), a drug in class B (beta blockers), a drug in class C (calcium channel blockers), and a drug in class D (diuretics), alone or in combination. In hypertensive emergencies, special drugs are used. Drugs in classes A and B are used for heart attacks, and drugs in classes A, B, and D are used for heart failure. Amiodarone is the most effective drug for arrhythmias. Drugs that inhibit platelet aggregation (acetylsalicylic acid and clopidogrel) or blood clotting (rivaroxaban and warfarin) are used for heart attacks and strokes. Lipid-lowering drugs such as simvastatin are used to prevent arteriosclerosis. Two risk factors for cardiovascular diseases are diabetes and tobacco smoking.

5.1 High Blood Pressure

Summary

High blood pressure (hypertension) is common. Without treatment, it leads to secondary diseases such as strokes, heart attacks, and heart failure. High blood pressure is treated with regular physical activity, a healthy diet, abstinence from tobacco use, and drug therapy. Drugs in class A (inhibitors of the renin–angiotensin–aldosterone system [RAAS]), drugs in class B (beta blockers), drugs in class C (calcium channel blockers), and drugs in class D (diuretics) can be combined to normalize blood pressure in almost all patients. Modern antihypertensive drugs are well tolerated and cause only mild adverse drug reactions (ADRs). The patient can contribute to the success of therapy by regular blood pressure checks.

Memo

- The basis of high blood pressure treatment is an active lifestyle with a healthy diet.
- Blood pressure control prevents secondary diseases.
- Modern high blood pressure therapy is effective and safe.
- Use of combinations of drugs in classes A, B, C, and D can reduce high blood pressure.
- Use of combinations of drugs in classes A and D can preserve the potassium balance.
- Drugs in class B lower the heart rate, cause cold fingers, and increase the risk of asthma attacks.
- Drugs in class C can cause dizziness and water retention in the lower legs.
- Potassium excess lowers the heart rate; potassium deficiency increases the heart rate.
- Never discontinue antihypertensives on your own; a hypertensive emergency may develop.

What Is High Blood Pressure?

When we talk about high blood pressure, we refer to high pressure in the arteries. Blood pressure is determined by two factors:

1. The cardiac workload
2. The resistance of the arteries

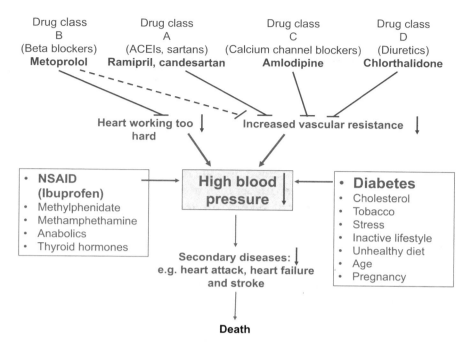

Fig. 5.1 How does high blood pressure develop, and how is it treated? In most patients, high blood pressure can be controlled with drugs in classes A, B, C, and D. Drugs in class A inhibit connective tissue remodeling processes in coronary heart disease and heart failure (see Sects. 5.2 and 5.3). Drugs in class B have an antiarrhythmic effect and protect the heart from overload in heart failure (see Sects. 5.2 and 5.3). To decrease blood pressure, the cardiac workload and/or the resistance of the arterial vessels must be reduced. Regular blood pressure checks can prevent secondary diseases. The most important risk factor for development of high blood pressure is diabetes (see Sect. 6.1). Various drugs can increase blood pressure. The most prominent example is excessive use of nonsteroidal anti-inflammatory drugs (NSAIDs; see Fig. 2.2)

If one or both factors are elevated, blood pressure rises. Figure 5.1 shows the development of high blood pressure, risk factors, therapeutic targets, and drugs that can aggravate high blood pressure.

Blood pressure is measured with a blood pressure cuff. The readings are expressed as the height of a mercury column in millimeters (mmHg). Two blood pressure values are determined: the systolic value (the upper reading) measures the heart's workload, and the diastolic value (the lower reading) measures the resistance of the arteries. Blood pressure should not be higher than 120/80 mmHg. If the upper reading is consistently higher than 140 mmHg and/or the lower reading is higher than 90 mmHg, the patient is diagnosed with high blood pressure. As blood pressure fluctuates during the day, 24-hour blood pressure measurement is often carried out to confirm the diagnosis.

In most cases, the exact cause of high blood pressure is unknown. This is obscured rather than explained by the terms "primary" or "essential" high blood pressure. The much rarer "secondary" forms of high blood pressure are caused by kidney disease or disease of the adrenal glands.

How Do I Know I Have High Blood Pressure?

Especially at the early stages, no symptoms are observed. The only way to make a diagnosis is to measure blood pressure regularly. In the doctor's office, however, blood pressure is often higher than normal because of anxiety. That's why you should measure your blood pressure at home. Easy-to-use devices are available. Sometimes high blood pressure manifests with nonspecific symptoms such as headaches, palpitations, or dizziness.

What Are the Consequences of Untreated High Blood Pressure?

Untreated high blood pressure leads to long-term damage to the arteries, which can impair the function of any organ. Particularly dangerous secondary diseases are heart attacks, heart failure, strokes, and kidney failure (see Sects. 5.2 and 5.3). Changes in retinal vessels may cause visual disturbances (see Sect. 10.2). Erectile dysfunction is a common complication and is often the first reason why a man with high blood pressure sees a doctor (see Sect. 7.2).

What Are the Risk Factors for Developing High Blood Pressure?

Untreated diabetes is the most important risk factor for high blood pressure (see Sect. 6.1). Other risk factors are elevated blood cholesterol levels (see Sect. 5.2), obesity, tobacco smoking, lack of exercise, an unhealthy diet, pregnancy, advanced age (women older than 65 years, men older than 55 years), and stress. Therefore, effective treatment of diabetes and high cholesterol—as well as a healthy lifestyle, with regular and moderate physical activity—reduces blood pressure. During pregnancy, blood pressure must be measured regularly.

High blood pressure can be worsened by drugs. A prime example are non-steroidal anti-inflammatory drugs (NSAIDs; see Sects. 2.1 and 11.2). These drugs inhibit the enzyme cyclooxygenase, which is particularly active in inflamed tissues. Cyclooxygenase generates prostaglandins that are important for kidney function. If cyclooxygenase is inhibited by NSAIDs, kidney function deteriorates. This leads to water retention (edema). The kidneys attempt to normalize their function by activating the renin–angiotensin–aldosterone system (RAAS), which causes blood pressure to rise. NSAIDs are dangerous if used long term (see Sects. 2.1 and 11.2). Avoid long-term use of NSAIDs!

An overdose of thyroid hormones (see Sect. 6.2) can increase blood pressure. Methylphenidate (see Sect. 9.1), which is used to treat attention deficit–hyperactivity disorder (ADHD), often causes high blood pressure in children and adolescents. Stimulant drugs such as methamphetamine and anabolic steroids, which are abused to build up muscles, can raise blood pressure. Thus, an essential factor in treatment of high blood pressure is avoidance of risk factors and harmful drugs.

Which Drugs Are Used for High Blood Pressure?

If it is not possible to normalize blood pressure by avoiding risk factors and taking general measures, treatment with antihypertensives must be initiated. Drug therapy is inexpensive because many generic drugs are available (see Sect. 1.2). Timely blood pressure reduction with antihypertensive drugs can prevent secondary diseases (see Sects. 5.2, 5.3, and 7.2) and maintain a high quality of life.

Modern antihypertensives reduce blood pressure effectively. They can be conveniently taken once a day, usually in the morning. This increases adherence to treatment considerably. For doctors, pharmacists, and patients to realize that blood pressure control is "child's play", antihypertensives are divided into drug classes A, B, C, and D. Drugs in classes A and B are additionally used for coronary heart disease (CHD; see Sect. 5.2), and drugs in classes A, B, and D are used for heart failure (see Sect. 5.3).

Table 5.1 summarizes important properties of drugs in classes A–D. All classes can be combined with each other, so it is possible to find a suitable drug combination for most patients. Patience, consideration of concomitant diseases, and regular blood pressure checks are the keys to successful antihypertensive therapy. By keeping a diary, the patient realizes that the medication is working. This is particularly important when the patient feels "healthy".

Table 5.1 Overview of the most important drug classes used for treatment of high blood pressure

Drug class	Prototype drug	Mechanisms of action	Important adverse drug reactions (ADRs) and interactions
Drug class A: angiotensin-converting enzyme inhibitors (ACEIs)	Ramipril	Formation of angiotensin (which constricts blood vessels) is reduced; as a result, vascular resistance decreases	Reduced potassium excretion, necessitating combined treatment with a drug in class D; irritating cough; dangerous swelling in the head region; kidney malformations in embryos
Drug class A: angiotensin receptor blockers (ARBs, sartans)	Candesartan	Angiotensin receptor antagonism; the effect of angiotensin on blood vessels is inhibited by blockade of angiotensin receptors; as a result, vascular resistance decreases	Similar to those associated with ACE inhibitors but no irritating cough and no swelling in the head region
Drug class B: beta-1 blockers (beta-1 receptor antagonists, beta blockers)	Metoprolol	Inhibition of the effect of the stress hormone epinephrine on the heart by blockade of beta-1 receptors; reduced sympathetic activity and less renin release	Fatigue; decreased libido; erectile dysfunction; risk of cold fingers; shortness of breath; failure to detect hypoglycemia in patients with diabetes
Drug class C: calcium channel blockers of the long-acting dihydropyridine type	Amlodipine	Inhibition of calcium influx into vessels; as a result, vascular resistance decreases	Headaches; swelling of the lower legs

(continued)

Table 5.1 (continued)

Drug class	Prototype drug	Mechanisms of action	Important adverse drug reactions (ADRs) and interactions
Drug class D: diuretics (inhibitors of sodium/chloride transport)	Chlorthalidone	Reduction of vascular resistance through a mechanism that is not precisely known	Increased potassium excretion, necessitating combined treatment with a drug in class A; need to ensure that fluid intake is sufficient

Drug-specific word stems are shown in bold text. Drugs in classes A and B are additionally used in coronary heart disease (CHD; see Sect. 5.2). Drugs in classes A, B, and D are used in chronic heart failure (see Sect. 5.3)
ACE angiotensin-converting enzyme, *ADR* adverse drug reaction, *ARB* angiotensin receptor blocker, *CHD* coronary heart disease

Drug Class A

As mentioned above in the context of NSAIDs, the renin–angiotensin–aldosterone system (RAAS) plays an important role in blood pressure regulation. This role can be exploited in drug therapy. The key molecule in this system is the first messenger angiotensin (hence the abbreviation "A" in the term "drug class A"). Angiotensin binds to angiotensin receptors (see Sect. 1.4) in the arteries. Therefore, the arteries become narrow, vascular resistance increases, and blood pressure rises.

Drug class A is divided into two subclasses: the older angiotensin-converting enzyme inhibitors (ACEIs) and the newer angiotensin receptor blockers (ARBs). The international nonproprietary names (INNs) of ACE inhibitors are recognized by the suffix "_pril". The INNs of ARBs contain the suffix "_sartan", and these drugs are therefore called "sartans".

ACEIs inhibit conversion of angiotensin precursor molecules into active angiotensin. As a result, less active angiotensin is available. Sartans bind to angiotensin receptors and act as antagonists to prevent the effects of angiotensin (see Sect. 1.4). As a result, angiotensin can no longer constrict the vessels. ACEIs and sartans lower arterial resistance and thus blood pressure.

However, an important difference between the two subclasses should be noted. Unlike sartans, ACEIs inhibit breakdown of bradykinin, a mediator of inflammation. This may cause a short-term, harmless, and irritating cough, but it can occasionally cause dangerous swelling of the face, lips, mouth, and larynx, which can impair breathing. If a patient treated with an ACEI notices swelling in their head region and shortness of breath, an emergency doctor must be called!

Because of these ACEI-specific ADRs, sartans are used in initial treatment of high blood pressure. If a patient has been treated with an ACEI for a long time without problems, this medication does not have to be switched. With use of a drug in class A, an effective and well-tolerated reduction in blood pressure can usually be achieved. The most important ADR associated with ACEIs and sartans is reduced excretion of potassium from the body (hyperkalemia [excess potassium]). This can lead to fatigue and a slowed heart rate (bradycardia). For this reason, the doctor regularly checks the potassium concentration (the "potassium level") in the blood. To prevent hyperkalemia, a drug in class A is usually combined with a drug in class D. This is an important example of a useful drug combination. Drugs in class A should not be given during pregnancy, because they can cause kidney malformations in the embryo.

Drug Class B

Binding of the stress hormone epinephrine (adrenaline) to beta-1 receptors in the heart leads to an increased workload and thus higher blood pressure. The effect of epinephrine is blocked by drugs in class B (beta blockers; see Sect. 1.4). Beta blockers not only reduce the cardiac workload but also decrease release of renin, which produces an angiotensin precursor (see above). Hence, beta blockers ultimately reduce the amount of active angiotensin. It takes about 1–2 weeks for a drug in class B to achieve an effective reduction in blood pressure.

Beta blockers, which are divided into nonselective beta blockers and selective beta-1 blockers, can be recognized by the drug-specific suffix "_olol" in their INNs. In the past, the nonselective beta blocker propranolol was commonly used to treat high blood pressure. However, because it was associated with ADRs affecting sugar metabolism (causing a risk of unrecognized hypoglycemia) and the respiratory tract (causing a risk of asthma attacks), propranolol is no longer used to treat high blood pressure.

The key to successful blood pressure lowering with a selective beta-1 blocker is to start with a low daily dose and increase it every 2 weeks until an adequate effect is achieved. If the effect is too small or if an ADR occurs, combination with other types of antihypertensive drugs can be useful.

Beta-1 blockers may cause fatigue, may reduce the libido, and, in men, may cause erectile dysfunction (see Sect. 7.2). If problems with the libido and erections occur, the patient should inform the doctor. In high doses, beta-1 blockers may cause dyspnea in patients with chronic obstructive pulmonary disease (COPD) or asthma (see Sects. 4.1 and 4.2), mask symptoms of hypoglycemia in patients with diabetes (see Sect. 6.1), and cause the fingers to become cold, white, and painful (Raynaud syndrome). These ADRs are mediated through blockade of the effects of epinephrine at beta-2 receptors. It is therefore important to be aware of these symptoms and to report them to your doctor. By reducing the dose, it should be possible to get these problems under control.

Drug Class C

In blood vessels, calcium channels mediate influx of calcium into muscle cells (see Sect. 1.4). Calcium triggers vasoconstriction and thus an increase in blood pressure. Calcium channel blockers (drug class C) prevent influx of calcium into muscle cells, dilate vessels, and thus lower blood pressure. In antihypertensive therapy, long-acting calcium channel blockers of the dihydropyridine type are used. They are recognized by the suffix "_dipine" in their INNs. The prototype drug is amlodipine, which provides a long-lasting and well-tolerated reduction in blood pressure. Nifedipine is a short-acting dihydropyridine. Because it causes fluctuations in blood pressure, it is no longer used in long-term therapy.

The main ADRs caused by long-acting dihydropyridines are due to their vasodilatory effects. Bilateral headaches (not to be confused with unilateral migraines) and water retention in the lower legs (not to be confused with signs of heart failure; see Sect. 5.3) may occur.

Drug Class D

The "D" in this class name stands for "diuretics". Beside its diuretic effect, this drug class has an antihypertensive effect: a reduced response to vasoconstrictive stimuli, which lowers vascular resistance. Chlorthalidone is the prototype drug in class D. In contrast to the drug classes A, B, and C, drugs in class D cannot be identified by a common suffix in their names. This is because these drugs have been around for decades and, in the past, during drug development, little thought was given to the importance and usefulness of systematic drug nomenclature (see Sect. 1.2). Drugs in class D have a slow onset of action, are effective, and are usually well tolerated.

The most important ADR associated with drugs in class D is increased excretion of potassium from the body (hypokalemia [low potassium]), which can be experienced as palpitations and nervousness. Drugs in class D are often combined with drugs in class A to avoid potassium problems.

Since drugs in class D promote excretion of water and sodium, care should be taken to ensure sufficient intake of fluids (e.g., mineral water and tea). A good fluid balance can easily be recognized when, after you squeeze the skin of your forearm with two fingers, no wrinkles remain and the skin returns to its original position quickly and is firm. The fluid requirement varies individually and is often overrated. Hyperhydration is more difficult to treat than dehydration.

How Is High Blood Pressure Treated During Pregnancy?

During pregnancy, high blood pressure can occur for the first time or existing high blood pressure can worsen. Both cases must be treated, otherwise the situation may develop into a hypertensive emergency, which can endanger the life of both the mother and the child. Drugs in class A have harmful effects on fetal development. Accordingly, a woman of childbearing age who is treated with a drug in class A must ensure safe contraception. If the patient wishes to become pregnant, the medication must be changed before pregnancy occurs. Drugs in classes B and D can be safely used during pregnancy. Methyldopa, which is otherwise rarely used because it causes fatigue, is considered safe in pregnancy.

Hypertensive Emergencies

A hypertensive emergency is an acute blood pressure derailment with diastolic readings (the lower of the two blood pressure numbers) above 120 mmHg and danger to life from a heart attack or cerebral bleeding. Pulsating headaches, visual disturbances, nosebleeds, nausea, and vomiting can point to a hypertensive emergency. The diagnosis is confirmed by blood pressure measurement.

The most frequent causes of a hypertensive emergency are inadequate long-term antihypertensive therapy and drug discontinuation by the patient. It is therefore important that the patient honestly reports any ADR, so that different drugs can be found if necessary.

If a hypertensive emergency is diagnosed by the patient themselves or by a relative, an emergency doctor must be called immediately. Until the doctor arrives, the patient should sit upright so that congestion of blood in the head is avoided. If the patient has glycerol trinitrate spray (see Sects. 2.1, 5.2, and 7.2) at hand, one or two puffs (but not more) can be administered. This can lower blood pressure and help to bridge the time until the emergency doctor arrives. The doctor will have a wider range of drugs available to decrease blood pressure and will arrange for the patient to be admitted to hospital.

5.2   Heart Attacks and Strokes

Summary

Heart attacks and strokes have common causes. High blood pressure, diabetes, high low-density lipoprotein (LDL) cholesterol levels, and tobacco consumption lead to arteriosclerosis. As a result, platelets aggregate (clump together) and blood vessels get clogged. The resulting lack of oxygen causes living tissue to die. It is therefore crucial to treat high blood pressure, high cholesterol, and diabetes. Effective and well-tolerated drugs are available for this purpose. Platelet aggregation can be inhibited with acetylsalicylic acid (ASA) in low doses and with adenosine diphosphate (ADP) receptor antagonists. Factor Xa inhibitors and vitamin K antagonists are used to inhibit blood clotting. An additional important risk factor for strokes is atrial fibrillation. It can be treated with amiodarone.

Memo

- Statins lower LDL cholesterol effectively; muscle pain is a warning sign of a statin overdose.
- In low doses, acetylsalicylic acid inhibits platelet clumping and prevents heart attacks and strokes.
- The most important ADR associated with acetylsalicylic acid is gastrointestinal bleeding.
- ADP receptor antagonists such as clopidogrel are an alternative to acetylsalicylic acid.
- Factor Xa inhibitors and vitamin K antagonists inhibit blood clotting with similar efficacy.
- Drugs in classes A and B prevent heart attacks.
- Atrial fibrillation can be treated with the antiarrhythmic drug amiodarone; many ADRs and interactions must be considered.
- Patients with a history of a heart attack or a stroke should avoid coxibs.

How Do Heart Attacks and Strokes Occur?

As heart attacks and strokes have similar causes, they are discussed together here. In these diseases, the arteries, which ensure the blood supply, get clogged. In a heart attack (myocardial infarction), the function of the heart is impaired and heart failure may occur (see Sect. 5.3). In the case of a stroke, paralysis of the arm and leg on one side, speech disturbance, and visual disturbance may occur. It is important to prevent heart attacks and strokes from the outset.

Figure 5.2 shows the development of myocardial infarction and strokes, and the targets of drug therapy. Arterial occlusion in these diseases is caused by three factors:

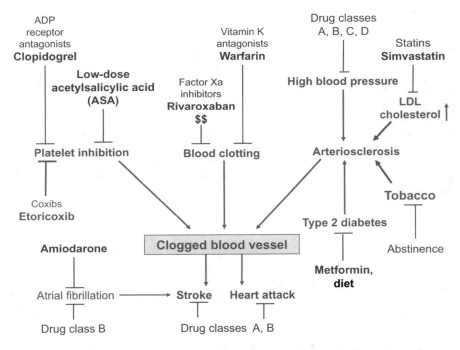

Fig. 5.2 How do heart attacks and strokes occur, and how are they treated? Heart attacks and strokes are caused by arterial occlusion. The occlusion is due to arteriosclerosis, which in turn is promoted by high blood pressure (see Sect. 5.1) and type 2 diabetes (see Sect. 6.1). Other risk factors are high low-density lipoprotein (LDL) cholesterol and tobacco use. For treatment of myocardial infarction and strokes, many more drug classes must be used than are needed for high blood pressure (see Fig. 5.1). Adverse drug reactions (ADRs) and drug interactions are correspondingly more serious. Avoid cyclooxygenase-2 inhibitors (coxibs). They can promote heart attacks and strokes. In many countries, factor Xa inhibitors (rather than vitamin K antagonists) are preferentially prescribed for strokes and myocardial infarction; this is a result of clever marketing and imposes a large financial burden on health care systems. (This figure does not show the treatment of myocardial infarction or coronary heart disease with stents that reopen clogged coronary arteries [see Table 5.2])

1. Arteriosclerosis (vascular calcification), based on chronic inflammation of the inner walls of blood vessels
2. Increased blood clotting
3. Platelet clumping

Arteriosclerosis is promoted by four major factors:

1. Diabetes
2. High blood pressure
3. High cholesterol
4. Tobacco consumption

Drugs as Risk Factors

Arteriosclerosis is associated with damage to the inner lining (endothelium) of arteries. As a result, platelets clump together and blood clotting is initiated. Heart attacks are caused by occlusion of coronary arteries. Strokes are often caused by blot clots (thrombi) transported from the left atrium of the heart to the brain. Blot clots in the left atrium are caused by disordered contraction of the atria. This dysfunction is called atrial fibrillation and is the most common cardiac arrhythmia. Strokes can also be caused by arteriosclerosis of the carotid arteries (neck arteries) and cerebral arteries.

It is important to avoid drugs that increase the risk of vascular occlusion. Among these drugs are coxibs (the prototype drug is etoricoxib). These drugs are advertised as a "stomach-friendly" alternative to NSAIDs (see Sect. 2.1), but they increase the risks of heart attacks and strokes. Therefore, patients with cardiovascular diseases must never take coxibs. Long-term treatment with coxibs (e.g., to relieve joint pain caused by osteoarthritis of the hip or knee) is particularly risky.

Certain antipsychotic drugs (see Sect. 9.4) can increase cholesterol levels and thus promote vascular occlusion. It is therefore necessary to check whether the doses of these drugs can be reduced or whether they can be replaced by alternatives that do not pose this risk.

How Are Heart Attacks and Strokes Treated?

This section discusses long-term treatment of myocardial infarction and strokes; it does not discuss acute therapy, which should take place under intensive care conditions. Table 5.2 summarizes the properties of important drug classes used for treatment of myocardial infarction and strokes.

Table 5.2 Overview of important drug classes used for treatment of myocardial infarction and strokes

Drug class	Prototype drug	Mechanisms of action	Indications	Important adverse drug reactions (ADRs) and interactions
Adenosine diphosphate (ADP) receptor antagonists	Clopido**grel**	Inhibition of platelet aggregation	Secondary prevention of strokes and heart attacks (*not* to be used for primary prevention)	Prolonged bleeding time and higher bleeding risk, particularly when combined with acetylsalicylic acid (ASA); treatment with ADP receptor antagonists is more expensive than treatment with ASA
Antiarrhythmics	Amiodarone	Blockade of various ion channels in the heart	Atrial fibrillation, ventricular tachycardia	Hypothyroidism or hyperthyroidism, photosensitivity, visual disturbances, pulmonary dysfunction, nerve damage, increased effect of warfarin (a vitamin K antagonist) by inhibition of its degradation; this is a clinically important interaction!
Factor Xa inhibitors (direct oral anticoagulants [DOACs], new oral anticoagulants [NOACs], xabans)	Rivaroxaban	Direct (rapid) inhibition of blood clotting factor Xa	Atrial fibrillation, heart attacks	Bleeding; factor Xa inhibitors have a faster effect and fewer interactions than vitamin K antagonists; significantly higher therapy costs; caution: since the duration of drug action is shorter than that of vitamin K antagonists, these tablets must be taken regularly, otherwise there may be no drug effect

Drug class	Prototype drug	Mechanisms of action	Indications	Important adverse drug reactions (ADRs) and interactions
Irreversible cyclooxygenase (COX) inhibitors	Acetylsalicylic acid (ASA)	Inhibition of platelet aggregation with a low dose (between one-tenth and one-fifth of the dose required for pain relief and inhibition of inflammation)	Secondary prevention of heart attacks and strokes (not to be used for primary prevention)	Prolonged bleeding time and higher risk of bleeding, especially in combination with ADP receptor antagonists; much less expensive than treatment with ADP receptor antagonists
3-Hydroxy-3-methylglutaryl coenzyme A (HMG-CoA) reductase inhibitors (statins, lipid-lowering agents, cholesterol-lowering agents)	Simvastatin	Inhibition of cholesterol formation in the liver, thereby lowering low-density lipoprotein (LDL) cholesterol	Secondary prevention of heart attacks and strokes in patients with hypercholesterolemia	Muscle soreness without physical loading, reddish urine, kidney failure (especially at high doses), interactions with other drugs that are broken down in the liver

(continued)

Table 5.2 (continued)

Drug class	Prototype drug	Mechanisms of action	Indications	Important adverse drug reactions (ADRs) and interactions
Vitamin K antagonists	Warfarin	Reduced formation of different clotting factors in the liver, leading to a delayed onset of action; blood clotting inhibition	Secondary prevention of strokes and heart attacks; despite aggressive advertising, there is *no need* to switch to a new oral anticoagulant (NOAC) if clotting is well controlled by a vitamin K antagonist	Increased risk of bleeding, hair loss, osteoporosis, numerous interactions with other drugs that are broken down in the liver (amiodarone is particularly crucial), numerous interactions with food; patients can make an important contribution to drug safety by monitoring their international normalized ratio (INR) value and adjusting their warfarin dose by themselves

Drug-specific word stems are shown in bold text. Drug classes A and B are discussed in Sect. 5.1
ADP adenosine diphosphate, *ADR* adverse drug reaction, *ASA* acetylsalicylic acid, *COX* cyclooxygenase, *DOAC* direct oral anticoagulant, *HMG-CoA* 3-hydroxy-3-methylglutaryl coenzyme A, *INR* international normalized ratio, *LDL* low-density lipoprotein, *NOAC* new oral anticoagulant

An important treatment option for coronary heart disease and heart attacks is insertion of stents into clogged coronary arteries. Stents open blood vessels from the inside, thereby improving blood flow. Stents are usually inserted with a catheter through an inguinal artery. This is a minimally invasive procedure. However, patients with a stent must still be treated with drugs.

Primary and Secondary Prevention

The most effective strategy to prevent heart attacks and strokes is to avoid risk factors for them. A distinction is made between primary prevention (before the disease occurs) and secondary prevention (after the disease has occurred).

Primary prevention includes abstinence from tobacco products, an active lifestyle, and a healthy diet, which reduce the risk of high blood pressure and diabetes. Diabetes (usually type 2) is treated with dietary changes, an active lifestyle, and the drug metformin (see Sect. 6.1). High blood pressure is treated effectively with drugs in classes A, B, C, and D (see Sect. 5.1). Secondary prevention includes reduction of high cholesterol levels with statins, inhibition of platelet aggregation with low-dose acetylsalicylic acid and ADP receptor antagonists, and inhibition of blood clotting with vitamin K antagonists and factor Xa inhibitors.

Drugs in class A (ACE inhibitors and sartans) and drugs in class B (beta blockers) lower blood pressure effectively (see Sect. 5.1). In addition, drugs in these two classes have a direct effect on the heart: beta blockers improve the ratio between oxygen supply and oxygen consumption and thus reduce the risk of angina pectoris attacks and heart attacks. However, they are not effective in acute angina pectoris attacks, which are treated with nitroglycerin (glyceryl trinitrate). Drugs in class A prevent scar tissue formation after a heart attack, thereby improving the contractility of the heart.

A common risk factor for strokes is atrial fibrillation. The antiarrhythmic drug amiodarone can eliminate atrial fibrillation. Alternatively, beta blockers can be used. Beta blockers do not eliminate atrial fibrillation, but they slow the heart rate and thus reduce the risk of thrombus formation.

Drug classes A, B, C, and D are described in Sect. 5.1. Metformin, which is used to treat type 2 diabetes, is described in Sect. 6.1. In sections "Cholesterol-Lowering Drugs", "When Statins Aren't Enough", "Platelet Aggregation Inhibitors", "Vitamin K Antagonists", "Alternatives to Vitamin K Antagonists", and "Amiodarone", we discuss statins, platelet aggregation inhibitors (acetylsalicylic acid and ADP receptor antagonists), anticoagulants (factor Xa inhibitors and vitamin K antagonists), and the antiarrhythmic drug amiodarone, respectively. The various drug classes are used in individually tailored combinations for treatment of heart attacks and strokes.

Cholesterol-Lowering Drugs

A distinction is made between "healthy" HDL (high-density lipoprotein) and "lousy" LDL (low-density lipoprotein). An LDL cholesterol value of more than 4.0 mmol/L (155 mg/dL) in the blood is called hypercholesterolemia. The higher this value, the higher the risk of a heart attack or a stroke. Drug treatment is aimed at lowering LDL cholesterol, whereby the target value depends on risk factors. It should be below 1.8 mmol/L (70 mg/dL) in anyone who has type 2 diabetes or a history of a heart attack. HDL cholesterol should be above 0.9 mmol/L (35 mg/dL). Hypercholesterolemia is just one risk factor for heart attacks and strokes. Therefore, LDL cholesterol lowering is only one measure among others. Whereas dietary cholesterol reduction is firmly established in primary and secondary prevention, the efficacy of cholesterol-lowering drugs has been proven only in secondary prevention.

LDL cholesterol lowering is started with HMG-CoA (3-hydroxy-3-methylglutaryl coenzyme A) reductase inhibitors (the prototype drug is simvastatin). All drugs with this mechanism of action have the suffix "_statin" in their INNs, which is why this class of drugs is commonly referred to as statins. These drugs inhibit formation of new cholesterol in the liver. If cholesterol formation is inhibited, the liver ensures the supply of cholesterol to the body by taking up more LDL cholesterol from the blood into the liver. As a result, the amount of LDL cholesterol in the blood decreases and the risk of a heart attack or a stroke is lowered.

Since cholesterol lowering is a preventive treatment, there is enough time to find the right statin dose for each patient by regular blood tests. The extents to which various statins reduce the risks of death from heart attacks and strokes are comparable. Since cholesterol formation in the liver is most active at night, the statin should be taken in the evening.

Statins are well tolerated. However, in high doses, they can impair the function of skeletal muscles, which manifests as sore muscles. Look out for any muscle pain that is not the result of an over-exertion of the muscle. If this warning sign is ignored, it can lead to muscle cell breakdown and release of the muscles' oxygen-binding protein (myoglobin). Myoglobin is excreted by the kidneys in the urine and turns it reddish. If this symptom occurs, you must immediately stop taking the statin and see your doctor, because myoglobin can clog kidney tubules and lead to kidney failure. The first measure is to drink plenty of fluids (tea or mineral water) to dilute the myoglobin in your urine and prevent blockage of kidney tubules.

The risk of ADRs associated with statins is increased if other drugs that are broken down in the liver are taken at the same time. The fewer additional drugs you take and the lower the statin dose you need, the safer the statin is. Ultimately, treatment with statins requires a compromise between adequate LDL cholesterol reduction and absence of serious ADRs.

When Statins Aren't Enough

If it is not possible to lower LDL cholesterol sufficiently with statins, additional drug classes can be used. These include PPAR (peroxisome proliferator–activated receptor) alpha receptor agonists (fibrates; the prototype drug is fenofibrate), bile acid binders (the prototype drug is cholestyramine), and inhibitors of cholesterol absorption in the intestine (the prototype drug is ezetimibe). These drugs are used in relatively few patients because they have only moderate effects on LDL cholesterol and can cause ADRs. In severe cases of hypercholesterolemia, evolocumab may be used. This drug must be injected subcutaneously and is much more effective than statins in lowering LDL cholesterol. However, evolocumab is very expensive.

Platelet Aggregation Inhibitors

Inhibitors of platelet aggregation are used in secondary prevention of heart attacks and strokes. Acetylsalicylic acid is the classic drug with this effect. Acetylsalicylic acid irreversibly inhibits the enzyme cyclooxygenase. It is found in all body cells, including blood platelets. In platelets, cyclooxygenase forms the platelet-clumping tissue hormone thromboxane. A single dose of acetylsalicylic acid inhibits cyclooxygenase in platelets for their entire lifetime (about 1 week) in the blood because platelets cannot make new cyclooxygenase. This fact can be exploited by taking a low dose (75–125 mg) of acetylsalicylic acid once a day. As a result, an inhibitory effect on platelet aggregation without an analgesic or anti-inflammatory effect can be achieved. For the latter effect, doses five to ten times higher are required.

The main ADR in long-term treatment with acetylsalicylic acid is an increased risk of bleeding. It manifests in a prolonged bleeding time—after shaving or cutting injuries, for example. In addition, gastrointestinal bleeding may occur. For this reason, it is important to regularly determine the level of hemoglobin in the blood and to look for unnoticed blood loss in the gastrointestinal tract with a stool test (detection of red blood pigment in the stools; see Sect. 3.2).

Platelets possess a specific receptor for the first messenger ADP, which promotes platelet aggregation. Irreversible ADP receptor antagonists (the prototype drug is clopidogrel) switch off the function of this receptor in the platelets for the lifetime of the cells (about 1 week). Thus, the effectiveness of clopidogrel and related drugs (all with the drug name suffix "_grel") in inhibiting platelet clumping is like that of acetylsalicylic acid. The most important ADR associated with ADP receptor antagonists is bleeding. Acetylsalicylic acid may be combined with ADP receptor antagonists if the patient is at high risk of a heart attack or a stroke. This drug combination increases the risk of bleeding. These different risks must be weighed against each other. Treatment with ADP receptor antagonists is more expensive than treatment with acetylsalicylic acid.

Vitamin K Antagonists

Warfarin and phenprocoumon are prototypical vitamin K antagonists and inhibit formation of several clotting factors in the liver. (For the sake of simplicity, here only warfarin is further mentioned as a drug.) The mechanism of action of vitamin K antagonists means that there is some delay in both the onset and the cessation of their effects. It takes several days before inhibition of blood clotting is fully established, and it takes several days before the effect wears off after warfarin discontinuation. In atrial fibrillation, warfarin inhibits formation of thrombi in the atrium and thus reduces the risk of a stroke.

Each patient's warfarin dosage must be adjusted individually. This is done by determination of the international normalized ratio (INR) value in the blood. To prevent a stroke, this value should be between 2.0 and 3.0; in patients with mechanical heart valves, it should be between 2.5 and 3.5. The higher the INR value, the higher the risk of bleeding. In former times, the patient had to go to the doctor to determine the INR value. However, conveniently manageable devices for INR measurement at home are now available. This facilitates therapeutic monitoring and adherence to treatment, and it strengthens the patient's personal responsibility. The most important ADR associated with warfarin is bleeding. Warfarin must not be used in pregnancy, as it is harmful to the fetus.

If warfarin is taken without other drugs, blood clotting can be well managed. However, problems arise if the patient takes other drugs. Warfarin is broken down in the liver. Other drugs are broken down in the liver as well, and this can lead to interference between drugs. Breakdown of warfarin is inhibited by the antiarrhythmic drug amiodarone (see Sect. 1.5). If the patient takes warfarin and amiodarone, the effect of warfarin is increased. On the other hand, if a patient treated with warfarin is taking drugs that speed up liver metabolism (e.g., the antiepileptic drugs carbamazepine or phenytoin or the herbal antidepressant St. John's wort; see Sects. 8.2 and 9.2), the effect of warfarin is weakened. Drugs that inhibit breakdown of warfarin in the liver (besides amiodarone, these include certain antibiotics and immunosuppressants; see Sects. 1.5, 11.2, and 11.3) enhance the inhibitory effect of the vitamin K antagonist on blood clotting.

Warfarin interacts with foods. "Healthy" foods high in vitamin K (these include kale, spinach, chives, chickpeas, fennel, and brussels sprouts) reduce the effects of warfarin. Conversely, foods such as the herb woodruff and goji berries, which inhibit the breakdown of warfarin, enhance its effects. Consuming such foods in small amounts is unproblematic, but any high intake must be avoided.

Alternatives to Vitamin K Antagonists

Because of problems related to treatment with warfarin and its interactions with drugs and food, "new" oral anticoagulants (NOACs) were introduced in the early 2000s, which were supposed to be more controllable and more effective. These drugs do not influence formation of clotting factors in the liver; instead, they directly inhibit the function of certain clotting factors in the blood. For this reason, these drugs are additionally called direct oral anticoagulants (DOACs).

A prototype of this drug class is rivaroxaban, which inhibits the clotting factor Xa. Because their names contain the drug-specific word stem "_xa_", the factor Xa inhibitors are known as xabans. The advantage of NOACs/DOACs/xabans is that they have a shorter duration of action than vitamin K antagonists. This is particularly important, for example, when bleeding occurs. Countermeasures can be taken more quickly. In addition, the coagulation capacity of the blood can be increased more quickly in the case of surgical interventions with a risk of bleeding. This flexibility in therapy with DOACs is an advantage over vitamin K antagonists.

However, as a disadvantage, treatment with DOACs is more susceptible to adherence problems or absorption disturbances (e.g., diarrhea; see Sect. 1.5) than is the case with vitamin K antagonists. In addition, no simple blood test to monitor the DOAC level is available. The efficacy of vitamin K antagonists and DOACs is equivalent, but DOACs are much more expensive than vitamin K antagonists. A patient who is well treated with warfarin does not have to be switched to a DOAC.

Amiodarone

Of all antiarrhythmics, amiodarone is the most effective drug. It prolongs the life of patients with atrial fibrillation by preventing strokes. After heart attacks, amiodarone prevents the occurrence of life-threatening arrhythmias originating from the ventricles.

Unfortunately, amiodarone is not easy to handle. Amiodarone remains in the body for a long time (up to 3 months), which is why treatment is difficult to control if ADRs occur. Amiodarone is highly fat soluble and therefore is distributed into many organs. Thus, it can be deposited in the cornea of the eye and cause visual disturbances. Amiodarone increases sensitivity to ultraviolet (UV) light through its deposition in the skin; thus, good sun protection is necessary. Furthermore, lung dysfunction and nerve damage may occur. Amiodarone can cause both hyperthyroidism and hypothyroidism (see Sect. 6.2). Therefore, regular specialist checks of the function of the thyroid, eyes, skin, lungs, and nervous system are necessary during treatment with amiodarone.

Amiodarone inhibits breakdown of certain drugs in the liver (see Sect. 1.5), thereby increasing the effects of these drugs. Therefore, when amiodarone and warfarin are administered at the same time, the INR value must be monitored carefully and the warfarin dose must be lower than usual. Otherwise, severe bleeding may occur.

5.3   Chronic Heart Failure

Summary

Chronic heart failure is the inability of the heart to supply the organs with sufficient oxygen and nutrients. The resulting symptoms are poor physical and mental fitness, shortness of breath, and water retention. Drugs in classes A and B and mineralocorticoid receptor antagonists (MCRAs) reduce mortality in chronic heart failure by improving maladaptation of the heart. Drugs in class D reduce water retention. To avoid potassium excess caused by use of drugs in class A and MCRAs, these drug classes should be combined with drugs in class D. It is important to avoid drug classes that may adversely affect cardiac function, such as NSAIDs.

Memo

- Drugs in classes A and B and MCRAs reduce mortality in chronic heart failure.
- Drugs in class D (diuretics) reduce water retention.
- NSAIDs should be avoided in chronic heart failure because of their ADRs.
- The main risk of combining a drug in class A and an MCRA is potassium excess (hyperkalemia).
- Hyperkalemia decreases the heart rate and physical fitness.
- Potassium excess caused by combination of a drug in class A and an MRCA is counteracted by simultaneous administration of a drug in class D.

Chronic Heart Failure

Chronic heart failure is the inability of the heart to supply the organs with sufficient oxygen and nutrients. The consequences of reduced organ perfusion are reduced physical and mental fitness, fatigue, shortness of breath, and water retention (edema), especially in the lower legs and lungs. The severity of heart failure is divided into four stages. The most important symptom for the classification is shortness of breath. At the first stage, heart failure is not yet clinically apparent and can be detected only by cardiac ultrasound. At the second stage, the patient's fitness is impaired during moderate physical activity; at the third stage, it is impaired during light activity; and at the fourth stage, the patient experiences shortness of breath at rest.

Chronic heart failure is common. More than 10% of the population over 70 years of age suffer from it. Figure 5.3 shows the development of chronic heart failure and treatment options.

The most important cause of chronic heart failure is inadequately treated high blood pressure (see Sect. 5.1). A greater workload is demanded because the heart must pump the blood against increased vascular resistance. In the short term, this can be accomplished by activation of the sympathetic nervous system, but the heart is not capable of managing a high workload over a long period. It attempts to counter this deficiency by growing muscle cells (hypertrophy). However, enlarged muscle cells consume more oxygen. The growth of blood vessels in the heart muscle does not keep up, and in the long term, the heart becomes undersupplied with oxygen and nutrients. This weakens the fitness of the heart further. The consequences are shortness of breath, fatigue, and reduced physical and mental fitness. In addition, blood backs up in the legs and lungs. This manifests as water retention, which is particularly critical in the lungs because it further reduces oxygen uptake into the body and increases shortness of breath.

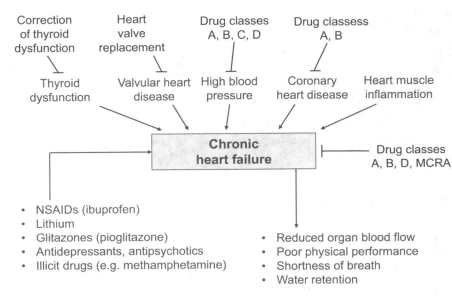

Fig. 5.3 How does chronic heart failure develop, and how is it treated? It is crucial to treat the causes of chronic heart failure, particularly high blood pressure (see Sect. 5.1) and thyroid disorders (see Sect. 6.2). Several drug classes can aggravate chronic heart failure. In treatment of chronic heart failure, drugs in classes A, B, and D are used. In addition, the MCRA drug class (mineralocorticoid receptor antagonists, aldosterone antagonists) is available. When a drug in class A and an MCRA are combined, the risk of hyperkalemia is high. This ADR is counteracted by administration of a drug in class D (Table 3.3)

As a result of heart failure, blood flow in the kidneys decreases. To compensate for this reduction, the kidneys release the hormones angiotensin and aldosterone. Angiotensin further constricts blood vessels and causes connective tissue growth in the heart, making it stiffer and less efficient. Aldosterone increases water retention and further increases heart stiffness.

Thus, chronic heart failure triggers a series of processes in the body that worsen the disease in a vicious cycle. Chronic heart failure is not curable. The mortality rate is comparable to those of many cancers (see Sect. 11.1). Terminal chronic heart failure can be successfully treated only by heart transplantation. However, because of the shortage of donor organs, many patients die from heart failure.

Underlying Diseases

An important cause of chronic heart failure is coronary heart disease (see Sect. 5.2), which can result from inadequately treated high blood pressure.

Coronary heart disease reduces the blood flow to the heart, which worsens heart failure. Coronary heart disease can be treated with drugs in classes A and B (see Sect. 5.2).

Chronic heart failure can be caused by thyroid dysfunction (see Sect. 6.2). Hyperthyroidism stimulates the sympathetic nervous system, thereby increasing blood pressure and the cardiac workload. This can lead to chronic heart failure. An underactive thyroid, on the other hand, weakens cardiac function in the long term as a result of the patient exercising too little.

The heart valves are essential for normal heart function. Therefore, heart valve defects can cause chronic heart failure in the long term. Heart valve defects are treated surgically whenever possible. Many valve defects can be corrected with minimally invasive surgery.

Another underestimated cause of chronic heart failure is myocarditis, which can be triggered by viral infections and often remains undetected. No causal treatment for viral myocarditis is available. The decisive factor is to avoid excessive physical activity to prevent life-threatening cardiac arrhythmias.

Problematic Drugs

Drugs can worsen heart failure. A prominent example of problematic drugs are NSAIDs, which are often used for long-term treatment of osteoarthritis (see Sect. 2.1). NSAIDs decrease blood flow in the kidneys and thereby worsen kidney function. Water retention is increased. Lithium, which has a mood-stabilizing effect (see Sect. 9.3), may reduce heart function and cause water retention. A patient with bipolar disorder and chronic heart failure must therefore be switched from lithium to another mood-stabilizing drug.

Until a few years ago, glitazones were touted as insulin-enhancing drugs (insulin sensitizers) in the treatment of type 2 diabetes. However, this euphoria has given way to disillusionment because glitazones can aggravate heart failure.

Many antidepressants and antipsychotics increase the heart rate by various mechanisms (see Sects. 9.2 and 9.4). This is unfavorable in chronic heart failure because the heart chambers (ventricles) cannot fill sufficiently. For this reason, antidepressants and antipsychotics must be dosed cautiously in patients with concomitant chronic heart failure.

Drug abuse can lead to heart failure. One of the most dangerous substances in this respect is methamphetamine (crystal meth), which activates the sympathetic nervous system. This can lead to an acute overload of the heart and consequently acute heart failure, especially if underlying diseases such as high blood pressure and coronary heart disease are present.

Heart Protection

Intuitively, the first two ideas for treating heart failure may be to (1) avoid physical activity and (2) strengthen your heart with drugs. These two treatment principles had been applied for decades until it became clear that avoiding physical activity and "strengthening" the heart with use of "cardiac glycosides" is counterproductive. Cardiac glycosides inhibit an enzyme (sodium/potassium ATPase) in every cell of the body. It is therefore predictable that "cardiac glycosides" cause a wide variety of ADRs. Nowadays, cardiac glycosides are obsolete. Table 5.3 summarizes the properties of drug classes used in treatment of chronic heart failure.

After these disappointing results, the following lesson was learned: instead of focusing on "heart strengthening", drug development focuses on correcting the body's maladaptation in heart failure, and this approach ("heart protection") is much more successful.

Eliminate Causes and Exercise as Best You Can

The most important aspect in chronic heart failure is to treat the underlying diseases. Treatment of high blood pressure is simple (see Sect. 5.1). With use of combinations of drugs in classes A, B, C, and D, almost any high blood pressure can be normalized. Treatment of coronary heart disease is more complicated (see Sect. 5.2). It is equally important to restore normal thyroid function. Hyperthyroidism is treated with thionamides, and hypothyroidism is treated with levothyroxine (see Sect. 6.2). Patients with chronic heart failure must avoid all drugs that could worsen their disease (see Fig. 5.3).

A second aspect in the treatment of chronic heart failure is to exercise the heart and the musculoskeletal system as best you can. This reduces the risk of acute heart failure. Appropriate physical training for chronic heart failure at stages 1–3 reduces mortality. Mild endurance activities such as cycling and walking are best.

Drugs for Heart Failure

Correction of the body's maladaptation represents the basis of drug treatment for chronic heart failure. MCRAs and drugs in classes A, B, and D are used. These drug classes can be combined according to the severity of heart failure. Combination therapy with an MCRA and drugs in classes A and B prolong

Table 5.3 Overview of drug classes used for treatment of chronic heart failure

Drug class	Prototype drug	Mechanisms of action	Important adverse drug reactions (ADRs) and interactions
Mineralocorticoid receptor antagonists (MCRAs, aldosterone antagonists)	Spironolactone	Inhibition of connective tissue growth in the heart, reduction of water retention	Potassium excess, especially in combination with a drug in class A; breast growth in men
Diuretics (drug class D, sodium/potassium/chloride cotransporter inhibitors)	Furo**semide**	Diuretic effect, blood pressure reduction	Potassium depletion, dehydration of the body, hearing damage; therefore, a combination of a drug in class A and an MCRA is used

Drug-specific word stems are shown in bold text. Drug classes A and B and the diuretic chlorthalidone are discussed in Sect. 5.1. During treatment of chronic heart failure, the potassium balance must be checked regularly. Both potassium excess and potassium deficiency are dangerous
ADR adverse drug reaction, *MCRA* mineralocorticoid receptor antagonist

life in chronic heart failure. Use of a drug in class D does not prolong life but does improve the quality of life.

Drugs in class A reduce the effects of angiotensin and delay connective tissue remodeling in the heart. They improve organ perfusion. The most important ADR associated with drugs in class A is potassium excess (hyperkalemia). It can slow down the heart rate and lead to fatigue. Hence, regular potassium monitoring is necessary. Potassium excess can be avoided if a drug in class A is combined with a drug in class D (a diuretic). Further properties of drugs in class A are described in Sect. 5.1.

Drugs in class B (beta blockers; the prototype drug is metoprolol) protect the heart from excessive stimulation by the sympathetic nervous system and thus prevent work overload. In Sect. 5.1, further properties of drugs in class B are discussed.

MCRAs reduce the harmful effects of the mineralocorticoid aldosterone on connective tissue remodeling in the heart. The prototype of this drug class is spironolactone. As with drugs in class A, the most important ADR associated with MCRAs is potassium excess. MCRAs and drugs in class A are often combined. In this case, the risk of potassium excess is high, and it is important to check the potassium level regularly.

The MCRA spironolactone is an antagonist not only at mineralocorticoid receptors, but also at receptors for the male sex hormone testosterone (androgen receptors). Therefore, men may experience breast enlargement (gynecomastia). If this is cosmetically disturbing, a switch to the MCRA eplerenone can be made. This drug has no antagonistic effect at androgen receptors. The reason why eplerenone is not routinely prescribed is that is more expensive than spironolactone.

The problem of high potassium can be controlled by adding a drug in class D (a diuretic) when using a drug in class A, an MCRA, or especially a class A + MCRA combination. Thiazide diuretics (the prototype drug is chlorthalidone) have a weaker effect on potassium excess than loop diuretics (the prototype drug is furosemide). The latter are effective in impaired kidney function. Thiazide diuretics and loop diuretics are often combined. Another important effect of diuretics is that they promote excretion of water and sodium chloride through the kidneys, thus reducing edema. However, although use of diuretics in chronic heart failure improves the quality of life, it does not increase the life expectancy. Thiazide diuretics are primarily used in long-term treatment of high blood pressure and are described in more detail in Sect. 5.1.

6

Drugs for Metabolic Disorders

Abstract This chapter discusses diabetes, thyroid diseases, and osteoporosis Type 1 diabetes is caused by insulin deficiency and is treated with insulin. The insulin dose is dependent on caloric intake and physical activity. The greatest danger is hypoglycemia; thus, patients with type 1 diabetes must carry glucose with them. Type 2 diabetes is caused by excessive caloric intake and physical inactivity. Correction of these two factors is the key to successful treatment. Metformin is the most effective drug in type 2 diabetes; it improves the overall metabolic situation. Hypothyroidism can be treated with levothyroxine. Hyperthyroidism is treated with inhibitors of thyroid hormone formation (thionamides) and a small amount of levothyroxine. Physical activity and adequate intake of calcium and vitamin D intake are crucial for treatment of osteoporosis. In severe osteoporosis, inhibitors of bone resorption (bisphosphonates and denosumab) can be used. These drugs can cause severe jaw damage; thus, prior dental restoration is important.

6.1   Diabetes

Summary

Diabetes comprises two different diseases. Type 1 diabetes patients lack the hormone insulin, which is responsible for absorption of blood glucose (sugar) into cells. This diabetes type is treated by a diet adapted to physical activity and administration of insulin in an appropriate dose. Hypoglycemia is a significant complication of type 1 diabetes. Therefore, patients with type 1 diabetes must carry glucose with them as an emergency treatment. Type 2 diabetes is due to excessive caloric intake, which causes the body to stop responding to insulin. As a result, the glucose concentration in the blood increases (hyperglycemia) and glucose is excreted in the urine. The most important measure for treatment of type 2 diabetes is a reduction in caloric intake. Metformin is the most effective drug for type 2 diabetes.

Memo

- Type 1 diabetes is characterized by insulin deficiency, which is treated with insulin.
- A complication of type 1 diabetes is hypoglycemia, which is treated with glucose.
- Alcohol consumption increases the risk of hypoglycemia.
- In type 2 diabetes, the body's sensitivity to insulin is reduced.
- The most effective treatment for type 2 diabetes is an active lifestyle and a healthy diet.
- Metformin is the most effective drug for treatment of type 2 diabetes.
- Use of metformin is safe if the contraindications for its use are considered.
- Metformin poses no risk of hypoglycemia.
- Gliptins, incretin mimetics, and gliflozins may be used if metformin is not effective enough.
- Certain antipsychotics and antidepressants can worsen diabetes.
- Treatment of diabetes complications such as high blood pressure, kidney failure, and nerve damage (polyneuropathy) is important.

How Does Diabetes Develop?

In diabetes, glucose (sugar) is excreted in the urine. Normally, the kidneys ensure that glucose remains in the body as the main source of energy. But if the concentration of glucose in the blood is too high (hyperglycemia), the kidneys are no longer able to retain the glucose completely. Excretion of

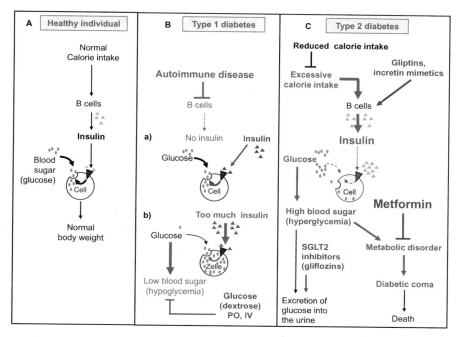

Fig. 6.1 How does diabetes develop, and how is it treated? **(a)** Healthy person. **(b)** Type 1 diabetes. **(c)** Type 2 diabetes. Insulin is produced in the B cells of the pancreas and causes uptake of glucose into cells. In type 1 diabetes, B cells are destroyed by an autoimmune disorder (see Sect. 11.2). Consequently, insulin is no longer produced. To compensate for this deficit, insulin must be administered. Insulins with different properties complement each other. The biggest problem with type 1 diabetes is hypoglycemia. It occurs when too much insulin is present in relation to glucose. Hypoglycemia is life threatening because the brain depends on glucose for its energy needs. Glucose must be administered if hypoglycemia is even only suspected. Type 2 diabetes is a different disease. Excessive caloric intake causes B cells to release large amounts of insulin. However, the insulin that is released no longer works, and the body becomes resistant to insulin. The result is hyperglycemia and serious metabolic derailment. A reduction in caloric intake is crucial in treatment of type 2 diabetes. The most effective drug for type 2 diabetes is metformin. It normalizes metabolic derailment. In addition, attempts can be made to increase insulin release with use of gliptins and incretin mimetics. Furthermore, hyperglycemia can be reduced by use of gliflozins to increase glucose excretion in the urine

glucose (glucosuria) is an early symptom of diabetes. A sweet urine odor and urinary tract infections (or vaginitis in women) may point to diabetes.

Two types of diabetes are distinguished. Figure 6.1 shows their development and treatment. In type 1 diabetes, B cells in the pancreatic islets are destroyed because of an autoimmune disease (see Sect. 11.2). B cells produce and release insulin. The most important task of insulin is to enable uptake of glucose into cells. Type 1 diabetes is caused by insulin deficiency. If insulin is lacking, the blood becomes hyperglycemic and then glucose is excreted in the urine (glucosuria). Although type 1 diabetes is an autoimmune disease, it is not treated with immunosuppressive drugs (see Sect. 11.2). Instead, insulin is replaced (see "How Is Type 1 Diabetes Treated?").

In type 2 diabetes, we have a completely different situation: the patient eats far too much, especially too much fat and sugar. B cells try to cope with the excessive caloric supply and secrete as much insulin as they can. Unfortunately, this is not a long-term solution, because, at the same time, the body cells become insensitive to insulin (insulin resistance). In other words, in type 2 diabetes, insulin is not missing; it just cannot work properly.

As a result, hyperglycemia and glucose excretion in the urine develop, as in type 1 diabetes. Often type 2 diabetes does not occur alone; it occurs together with other diseases, especially high blood pressure (see Sect. 5.1), high cholesterol (see Sect. 5.2), and obesity. This combination is known as metabolic syndrome.

Important risk factors for development of type 2 diabetes are a sedentary lifestyle and an unhealthy diet high in calories, fat, and sugar, especially consumption of sugary soft drinks (soda pop). The best prevention for type 2 diabetes is an active lifestyle and a healthy diet. A good biomarker for long-term management of diabetes is the amount of glucose attached to the oxygen carrier hemoglobin A_{1c} (HbA_{1c}).

How Is Type 1 Diabetes Treated?

The goal of treating type 1 diabetes is to achieve optimum metabolic control without hyperglycemia so that long-term complications such as high blood pressure, heart attacks, strokes, kidney failure (diabetic nephropathy), and nerve damage (diabetic polyneuropathy) are avoided. The principle of treating type 1 diabetes is to match caloric intake and insulin administration. There is no need for a reduction in caloric intake. You can do any physical activity, including competitive sports. It is crucial that you learn, through good nutritional counseling, how much insulin you need to supply for given amounts and types of food you eat.

Insulin must be injected subcutaneously. A distinction is made between short-acting and long-acting insulins. These types of insulin complement each other. Short-acting insulins are important for immediate utilization of nutrients from a meal, while long-acting insulins provide the basic supply of insulin for the body. Table 6.1 lists a short-acting insulin and a long-acting insulin

Table 6.1 Overview of the most important drug classes used for treatment of diabetes

Drug class	Prototype drug	Mechanisms of action	Indications	Important adverse drug reactions (ADRs) and interactions
Short-acting insulins	Insulin lispro	Increased glucose uptake into cells	Type 1 diabetes; to be injected under the skin 5–15 minutes before meals; duration of action: up to 3 hours	Hypoglycemia, lipodystrophy
Long-acting insulins	Insulin glargine	Increased glucose uptake into cells	Type 1 diabetes; basal insulin supply to the body; onset of action after 4 hours; duration of action: 24 hours	Hypoglycemia, lipodystrophy
Biguanides	Metformin	Improvement of metabolic derailment	Type 2 diabetes; clinical trials have shown a life-prolonging effect; gold standard in treatment of type 2 diabetes	Metallic taste, loss of appetite, nausea, vomiting, diarrhea; risk of lactic acidosis in patients at risk; no risk of hypoglycemia
Dipeptidyl peptidase 4 (DPP4) inhibitors (gliptins)	Sita**gliptin**	Increased effect of incretin hormones by inhibition of the enzyme DPP4, which is responsible for degradation of incretin hormones	Type 2 diabetes; add-on therapy if biguanide treatment does not suffice; not superior to biguanides	Gastrointestinal disturbances, respiratory infections, low risk of hypoglycemia

(continued)

Table 6.1 (continued)

Drug class	Prototype drug	Mechanisms of action	Indications	Important adverse drug reactions (ADRs) and interactions
Incretin receptor agonists (incretin mimetics)	Liraglutide	Activation of incretin receptors (as an agonist)	Type 2 diabetes; add-on therapy if biguanide treatment does not suffice; to date, not shown to be superior to biguanides	Gastrointestinal disturbances, low risk of hypoglycemia
Sodium/glucose cotransporter 2 (SGLT2) inhibitors (gliflozins)	Empa**gliflozin**	Reabsorption of glucose by the kidneys is inhibited by blockade of the transporter SGLT2; as a result, glucose is excreted in the urine	Type 2 diabetes; add-on therapy if biguanide treatment does not suffice; not superior to biguanides	Hypoglycemia, dehydration of the body (water deprivation), blood pressure drops, risk of vascular occlusion (thrombosis), increased risk of urinary tract infections (and, in women, vaginal infections), increased risk of osteoporosis

Drug-specific word stems are shown in bold text. Metformin is the oldest, least expensive, and most effective drug for treatment of type 2 diabetes. Despite strong promotion of newer diabetes drugs (gliptins, incretin mimetics, and gliflozins), metformin is the gold standard. The key to successful treatment of type 2 diabetes is a healthy diet and an active lifestyle, not drug therapy

ADR adverse drug reaction, DPP4 dipeptidyl peptidase 4, SGLT2 sodium/glucose cotransporter 2

as examples. Insulins that need to be injected only 5–15 minutes before eating are particularly suitable for a flexible and high-quality lifestyle.

In traditional therapy, a long-acting insulin is injected to ensure the body's basic supply of insulin. Additionally, a short-acting insulin is administered at mealtimes, the dose of which is adapted to the carbohydrate intake. In modern treatment regimens, the current blood glucose concentration is factored into dosing of insulin. Convenient small devices can be implanted under the skin and measure tissue glucose concentrations. The most accurate way to treat type 1 diabetes is with use of an insulin pump.

The most commonly used devices are insulin pens, which make injecting precise doses much easier and more convenient than conventional syringes. Most insulin pens contain 100 international units of insulin per milliliter (100 IU/mL). One click on the pen is equivalent to one unit of insulin. This allows you to adjust the insulin dose precisely for the amount of carbohydrates you eat.

Avoid storing insulin pens in direct sunlight or in a car. Exposure to heat will render the insulin ineffective. Your supply of insulin pens should be stored in a cool place, but be sure to avoid storing them in the freezer, because that causes the insulin to become inactive.

Avoid randomly changing insulin injection sites between different parts of the body, as this may alter the absorption of insulin into the body. Insulin is rapidly absorbed from abdominal fat, which is therefore a particularly suitable site for injection of short-acting insulins. On the other hand, insulin is absorbed slowly from the thigh, which is why you should inject mainly delayed-release insulins there. Within a given body region (e.g., abdominal fat), change the injection site by 1 cm each day. This is important for reliable insulin absorption.

If you do not take these precautionary measures, the fat tissue can harden and develop an orange peel texture (lipodystrophy). This is not only cosmetically disturbing but also painful. Above all, lipodystrophy delays absorption of insulin into the body. This leads to poorer metabolic control.

It is important that you use a new needle every day. Blunt needles increase the risks of infection and lipodystrophy. Follow the manufacturer's instructions for storing the insulin pens. Ideally, the pen you are currently using should be stored at room temperature.

Which Adverse Drug Reaction Can Occur with Insulin Treatment?

The flip side of the goal of avoiding hyperglycemia is an increased risk of hypoglycemia. Hypoglycemia is life threatening! Hypoglycemia (a blood glucose concentration lower than 50 milligrams per deciliter [50 mg/dL] or 2.8 millimoles per liter [2.8 mmol/L]) can occur because of too much physical activity, too little energy intake, too high an insulin dose, or a combination of these factors. Warning signs include palpitations, tremors, restlessness, and craving for sugar. As the brain depends on glucose as its main source of energy, confusion, seizures (see Sect. 8.2), and unconsciousness may occur. Hypoglycemia is confirmed by finger prick blood tests or bloodless measurement of glucose concentrations.

In emergency treatment of hypoglycemia, 15–30 grams (15–30 g) of glucose must be supplied immediately. Every patient with diabetes and every relative of a patient with diabetes must have glucose handy. If it is not possible to confirm the presence of hypoglycemia, administer glucose anyway if in doubt. Short-term hyperglycemia is harmless. Consumption of alcohol can aggravate hypoglycemia! The warning symptoms of hypoglycemia can be attenuated, especially by use of high-dose beta blockers for treatment of cardiovascular diseases.

What Do I Need to Consider When Dosing Insulin?

As a rule of thumb, the body needs 0.5–1 IU of insulin per kilogram of body weight (0.5–1 IU/kg) per day. Approximately 40% of this amount is for the basic supply (long-acting insulin) and 60% must be covered by short-acting insulin. The insulin requirement for a given amount of carbohydrate is highest in the morning; i.e., more insulin needs to be injected in the morning than at lunchtime, when the insulin requirement is lowest. If you are physically active, you will need less insulin than if you are inactive. Physical activity increases your body's sensitivity to insulin.

Care must be taken with various diseases and drugs that alter the body's sensitivity to insulin. Pregnancy, fever, infections, major surgery, and hyperthyroidism (see Sect. 6.2) increase insulin requirements, as does treatment with high doses of glucocorticoids in autoimmune diseases (see Sect. 11.2). Conversely, insulin requirements are reduced in hypothyroidism (see Sect. 6.2).

How Is Type 2 Diabetes Treated?

Treatment of type 2 diabetes can be derived from the origins of the disease. Since it is based on overeating and reduced insulin sensitivity, these two factors must be corrected.

The basis of therapy for type 2 diabetes is a healthy diet and an active lifestyle. Physical activity increases the insulin sensitivity of B cells and thus reduces the stress on them. If you, as a patient, are prepared to change your lifestyle, you will probably manage without drugs for type 2 diabetes. If lifestyle changes alone are not sufficient, treatment of type 2 diabetes can be supported by drugs. The most important drugs in question are discussed in sections "Metformin, the Gold Standard", "Gliptins and Incretin Mimetics", "Gliflozins", and "Other Drugs". Table 6.1 summarizes the properties of these drugs.

Metformin, the Gold Standard

Metformin is a biguanide. It was introduced into diabetes treatment almost 70 years ago. Metformin is the most effective and least expensive drug for treating type 2 diabetes. It improves metabolic derailment. One feature of metformin treatment is loss of appetite. This is desirable "biofeedback" because it reduces obesity. To date, metformin is the only drug for which a life-prolonging effect has been demonstrated in type 2 diabetes.

These are important arguments in favor of metformin because type 2 diabetes requires long-term therapy. Although metformin has been used for a long time in type 2 diabetes, its exact mechanism of action is still unknown. Originally, an improvement in the insulin sensitivity of cells (insulin sensitization) was thought to be decisive in the effect of metformin, but this cannot be the reason, as other insulin sensitizers (glitazones; the prototype drug is pioglitazone) do not have a life-prolonging effect.

The daily dose of metformin can be adjusted on the basis of the metabolism and tolerability. Moreover, unlike insulin, metformin can be taken in the form of tablets. The dose of metformin is increased gradually, depending on the effect and side effects. The maximum dose of metformin is 1 g three times per day.

Metformin does not increase body weight and poses no risk of hypoglycemia. In rare cases, metformin can cause lactic acidosis. Patients with chronic heart failure, liver failure, or kidney failure are particularly at risk. To minimize the risk, metformin should not be used in patients with these conditions. For safety reasons, metformin should not be used in patients with alcohol dependence, pancreatitis, cancer, or infectious diseases. If these contraindications of metformin are observed, it is a safe drug to use.

The main adverse drug reactions (ADRs) caused by metformin are nausea, vomiting, and diarrhea. In addition, patients occasionally complain of a metallic taste. In most cases, the ADRs decrease over time, with no reason to discontinue metformin if symptoms occur at the beginning of treatment.

Gliptins and Incretin Mimetics

One problem with type 2 diabetes is "stressed B cells", which cannot secrete enough insulin to compensate for the increased demand due to insulin resistance. In the past, sulfonylureas were used frequently. They increase the release of insulin. However, the disadvantage of these drugs is that the insulin release is independent of the actual glucose concentration in the blood. Because of the high risk of hypoglycemia, lack of a life-prolonging effect, and development of better-tolerated drugs, use of sulfonylureas has continuously decreased over the years.

Incretins stimulate release of insulin in B cells only if glucose is present. Therefore, the stimulation of insulin release by incretins is much more targeted than that of sulfonylureas. Currently, many hopes rest on treating type 2 diabetes with enhancers of the incretin system. Incretin enhancers pose a significantly lower risk of hypoglycemia than sulfonylureas.

We have two ways to enhance the incretin system. First, degradation of incretins can be inhibited. This is achieved by use of dipeptidyl peptidase 4 inhibitors (DPP4 inhibitors; the prototype drug is sitagliptin). Since the international nonproprietary names (INNs) of these drugs have the suffix "_gliptin", the drug class is called gliptins. The second way to enhance the incretin system is to attempt to directly stimulate incretin receptors (see Sect. 1.4), using incretin mimetics (incretin receptor agonists). To date, however, there is a lack of evidence that incretin enhancers are superior to metformin in long-term therapy. Therefore, their status is that of an add-on therapy for use with metformin.

Gliflozins

These drugs inhibit reuptake of glucose from urine into the kidneys and thus into the body through a transporter (sodium/glucose cotransporter 2 [SGLT2]; see Sect. 1.4). The INNs of all drugs in this class have the suffix "_gliflozin". As reabsorption of glucose into the body is decreased, hyperglycemia is improved and more glucose is excreted in the urine. However, as the urine becomes more nutrient-rich with gliflozin therapy, the risk of bacterial urinary tract infections increases, as does the risk of vaginal infections in women (see Sect. 11.3). Moreover, osteoporosis (see Sect. 6.3) and hypoglycemia may develop. There is still a lack of evidence that gliflozins are clinically superior to biguanides. For this reason, gliflozins are used as an add-on therapy in type 2 diabetes. Interestingly, gliflozins may have beneficial effects in heart failure and kidney failure.

Other Drugs

Until a few years ago, glitazones (insulin sensitizers) were popular in treatment of type 2 diabetes. However, use of these drugs has declined sharply because, in addition to a lack of a life-prolonging effect in type 2 diabetes, their use is associated with increased risks of weight gain, water retention, heart attacks, heart failure (see Sect. 5.3), and, in women, a higher risk of bone fractures (see Sects. 6.3 and 7.1).

Acarbose inhibits digestion of carbohydrates in the intestine. As a result, less glucose is absorbed into the blood. Unfortunately, the undigested carbohydrates are fermented in the colon by bacteria and cause intestinal cramps, flatulence, and diarrhea. Because of its poor tolerability and low efficacy, acarbose has little value in the treatment of type 2 diabetes.

Diabetes is a major risk factor for development of cardiovascular and kidney diseases. Therefore, simultaneous treatment of these diseases in patients with diabetes plays an important role (see Sects. 5.1–5.3). Drug class A (see Sect. 5.1) can be used to delay diabetic kidney damage (nephropathy). In type 2 diabetes, simultaneous treatment of cardiovascular disease (see Sects. 5.1–5.3), diabetic nephropathy, and dyslipidemia (see Sect. 5.2) is important.

In type 2 diabetes, insulin is used only at the late stages when the B cells are completely exhausted and unable to function. The danger here is that significant weight gain may occur.

Certain antidepressants and antipsychotics (see Sects. 9.2 and 9.4) may worsen type 2 diabetes. Therefore, these drugs should be used cautiously in patients with type 2 diabetes. If their use is essential, patients should be encouraged to adopt a healthy lifestyle.

6.2   Thyroid Diseases

Summary

The thyroid gland releases the hormone thyroxine. It influences almost all bodily functions. Both too much thyroid hormone (hyperthyroidism) and too little thyroid hormone (hypothyroidism) are unpleasantly noticeable. The main symptoms of hyperthyroidism are palpitations, high blood pressure, nervousness, trembling, sensitivity to heat, sweating, diarrhea, and weight loss. Hyperthyroidism is treated with inhibitors of thyroid hormone production (thionamides). In addition, the patient takes a small amount of thyroid hormone (levothyroxine [synthetic thyroxine], T4) to prevent thyroid enlargement from occurring. During this treatment, the blood count must be checked regularly. The main symptoms of hypothyroidism are a decrease in the heart rate, dizziness, fatigue, sensitivity to cold, dry skin, constipation, and weight gain. Hypothyroidism is treated with T4.

Memo

- Thyroid diseases can affect any organ.
- Consumption of iodized salt and marine fish prevents hypothyroidism.
- Self-observation of your body plays a key role in treatment of thyroid disease.
- Drugs for treatment of thyroid disease have a slow onset of action.
- Thionamides are used to treat hyperthyroidism.
- Thionamides can cause a drop in white blood cell numbers.
- Treatment of hypothyroidism with T4 must be precise.
- T4 must be taken in the morning on an empty stomach.
- You are strongly warned against taking "natural" thyroid hormones.

What Is the Task of the Thyroid Gland?

To better understand development of thyroid diseases and their treatment, it is necessary to explain the function of the thyroid gland. Figure 6.2 gives an overview of the symptoms of thyroid diseases and their treatment. In Table 6.2, the most important drug classes used for treatment of thyroid diseases are listed. The thyroid gland is a butterfly-shaped organ, which lies below the larynx. During swallowing, the thyroid gland moves upward. In a healthy person, the thyroid gland is barely visible.

The thyroid gland produces thyroid hormone. This hormone influences almost all bodily functions. Your body needs a certain amount of thyroid hormone to keep you physically and mentally fit. The thyroid gland stores

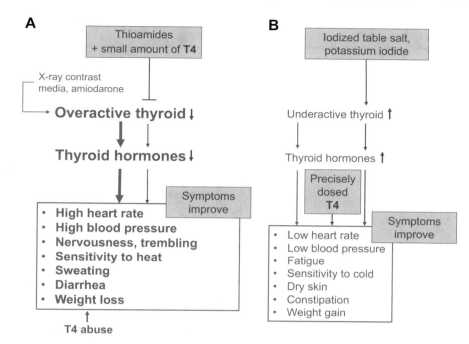

A

Thioamides + small amount of **T4**

X-ray contrast media, amiodarone

Overactive thyroid ↓

Thyroid hormones ↓

Symptoms improve

- **High heart rate**
- **High blood pressure**
- **Nervousness, trembling**
- **Sensitivity to heat**
- **Sweating**
- **Diarrhea**
- **Weight loss**

↑
T4 abuse

B

Iodized table salt, potassium iodide

Underactive thyroid ↑

Thyroid hormones ↑

Precisely dosed **T4**

Symptoms improve

- Low heart rate
- Low blood pressure
- Fatigue
- Sensitivity to cold
- Dry skin
- Constipation
- Weight gain

Fig. 6.2 How do thyroid diseases develop, and how are they treated? (a) Hyperthyroidism. (b) Hypothyroidism. In many cases, thyroid dysfunction is due to an autoimmune disease (see Sect. 11.2). Many symptoms of hyperthyroidism and hyperthyroidism are mirror images of each other and easily recognizable to patients affected by each disease. Thus, patients themselves can make an important contribution to optimal treatment. It is logical to treat an iodine deficiency with iodine and to treat a thyroid hormone deficiency with thyroid hormone (T4). What is a little more difficult to understand is why you need to take a small amount of T4 in addition to thiamazole (a thionamide) for hyperthyroidism. The reason is to prevent excessive growth of the thyroid gland and to ensure a basic supply of T4. A major problem is T4 abuse with the goal of weight loss. In addition, T4 can promote bipolar disorder (see Sect. 9.3)

some thyroid hormone for situations in which iodine supply is reduced. Therefore, changes in thyroid function are slow to manifest during both disease development and treatment. Therefore, observe your body carefully.

Thyroid disorders manifest themselves in many organs. They can lead to disturbed cardiovascular function and digestion, changes in skin and hair, sensitivity to heat or cold, and changes in body weight and mental state. Thyroid disease can be the cause of unwanted childlessness. It is a good idea to consider the possibility of a thyroid disease in the event of unclear bodily complaints that develop slowly.

Table 6.2 Overview of the most important drug classes used for treatment of thyroid diseases

Drug class	Prototype drug	Mechanisms of action	Indications	Important adverse drug reactions (ADRs) and interactions
Thionamides	Thia**mazole**	Inhibition of thyroid hormone formation (thyroid peroxidase inhibitor)	Hyperthyroidism; used in combination with a small amount of T4 to prevent thyroid enlargement	Mild and transient: rash, joint pain, nausea, vomiting; in about 0.5% of all patients, white blood cell numbers drop; therefore, blood cell count checks are required; risk of hypothyroidism in the event of an overdose
Thyroid hormones	Levothyroxine (T4): 75–125 µg/day in women, 125–200 µg/day in men	Inactive precursor; converted into active thyronine (T3) in the body	Hypothyroidism; add-on therapy for hyperthyroidism to prevent thyroid enlargement and ensure a basic thyroid hormone supply to the body	Hyperthyroidism in the event of an overdose, otherwise well tolerated; adjust the dose in the case of concomitant diseases; do not take together with iron preparations; risk of abuse for weight loss and muscle building
Iodized salt	Potassium iodide: 100–200 µg/day	Support of thyroid hormone synthesis	Hypothyroidism with a proven iodine deficit; mostly in iodine-deficient environments	Risk of hyperthyroidism in the event of an overdose

Drug-specific word stems are shown in bold text. Potassium iodide and T4 are dosed in the microgram (µg) range; 1 milligram (1 mg) is equivalent to 1000 µg. This dosing in the microgram range is rare for a drug and can cause overdosing. It is a misconception that "natural thyroid hormones" (often ill-defined mixtures of T3 and T4) work better and more safely than T4. Such preparations are dangerous

ADR adverse drug reaction, *mg* milligram, *T3* thyronine, *T4* levothyroxine, *µg* microgram

Thyroid hormone contains iodine atoms. The thyroid gland can absorb iodine from the blood and store it. Iodine is taken up from water and food. To ensure adequate intake of iodine for formation of thyroid hormone, use of iodized table salt is recommended. You should eat marine fish or other seafood at least once a week. In many alpine environments, the iodine supply is low. In these environments, adequate iodine intake is particularly important to prevent development of thyroid diseases.

If the iodine supply is too low and thus the formation of thyroid hormone is reduced, the thyroid gland tries to solve this problem. It starts to grow under the influence of a hormone (thyroid-stimulating hormone [TSH]) from the pituitary gland. However, this adaptation mechanism does not work properly, and so thyroid diseases can develop. The most common diseases in this context are hypothyroidism and a benign thyroid tumor (adenoma) or a malignant thyroid tumor (cancer). In addition, the thyroid gland "strangles" the larynx and the esophagus from the front, and, in addition to the cosmetic disfigurement caused by an enlarged thyroid gland (goiter), swallowing disorders may occur. Surgery is more difficult to perform on an enlarged thyroid gland than on a normal-sized thyroid gland.

How Do I Know I Have Hyperthyroidism?

In most cases, hyperthyroidism develops gradually. The reasons are as follows:

1. Thyroid hormone mediate changes in gene function through its receptors. This process is slow by nature (see Sects. 1.4, 4.1 and 11.2).
2. The thyroid gland stores a thyroid hormone supply for use in times of need.

If you have more than one of the following symptoms, you should see your doctor. The main symptoms of hyperthyroidism are a rapid heartbeat, high blood pressure, nervousness, restlessness, tremors, sensitivity to heat, sweating, diarrhea, and weight loss. In hyperthyroidism, the production of thyroid hormone is increased and causes the symptoms mentioned above. We distinguish between two major causes of hyperthyroidism:

1. Uncontrolled hormone production caused by an adenoma. An adenoma often develops because of thyroid enlargement in iodine-deficient environments.
2. An increase in thyroid hormone production due to an immune reaction directed against the body (autoimmune disease; see Sect. 11.3). The eyeballs often protrude, and the white part of the eye (sclera) is clearly visible. The technical term for bulging eyes is "exophthalmos".

How Is Hyperthyroidism Treated?

The aim of hyperthyroidism treatment is to eliminate all symptoms and restore normal body functions (euthyroidism). If possible, adenomas are removed surgically. If surgical therapy is not an option, hyperthyroidism is treated with drugs. Unlike other autoimmune diseases, hyperthyroidism caused by an autoimmune disease is not treated with immunosuppressive drugs (see Sect. 11.2). Instead, drugs that reduce thyroid gland function are used.

The most important class of drugs for treatment of hyperthyroidism are the thionamides (the prototype drug is thiamazole [methimazole]). Thionamides stop excess formation of thyroid hormone in the thyroid gland. Treatment with thionamides is easy to perform, as they only need to be taken once a day. The individual dose of the drug is adjusted according to the severity of hyperthyroidism.

Thionamides do not affect thyroid hormone release from the thyroid gland. First, the supply of stored thyroid hormone is used up before thionamides show a clinical effect, which might take 1–2 weeks. During this time, the patient must not interrupt the treatment on their own initiative even if they don't think it's working.

If you do not feel well between the start of treatment and the onset of the effects of thionamide, your doctor may prescribe drugs to treat certain symptoms in the short term. Beta-1 blockers can relieve palpitations and lower blood pressure (see Sect. 5.1). Benzodiazepines (see Sect. 8.2) can reduce nervousness but can be addictive; therefore, they should be used only with caution. Loperamide (see Sect. 3.3) can stop diarrhea. It is best to just wait, and not take other drugs, until the thionamide starts to work.

Therapy with thionamides is long-term, and regular drug intake is essential for successful therapy. Skin rashes, joint pain, nausea, and vomiting are common ADRs associated with thionamides but are usually transient and do not require discontinuation of therapy.

The most important and dangerous ADR associated with thionamides is a decrease in white blood cell numbers (agranulocytosis). It occurs, on average, in 0.5% of all patients. Therefore, your doctor must check your blood count regularly. Warning signs of a drop in white blood cell numbers can be a sudden fever, chills, and infections, including fungal infections in the mouth. See your doctor right away! Your doctor can detect a drop in your white blood cell numbers quickly with a blood count. If it is detected in time, the prognosis is good. Your doctor will discontinue use of the triggering drug. In addition, the hormone G-CSF (granulocyte colony–stimulating factor) is administered, which stimulates formation of white blood cells again.

Some drugs can trigger or aggravate hyperthyroidism. These include iodine-containing X-ray contrast media and amiodarone, which is effective in certain cardiac arrhythmias (e.g., atrial fibrillation; see Sect. 5.2). Thus, if you receive treatment from a radiologist or a cardiologist, it is important for you to inform them that you are being treated for hyperthyroidism.

Hyperthyroidism is never treated with thionamides alone. In addition, a small amount of thyroid hormone is given. At first glance, it may seem contradictory as to why more thyroid hormone is given in cases of hyperthyroidism. This is why:

1. The body needs a certain amount of thyroid hormone, otherwise hypothyroidism develops. The additionally given thyroid hormone is therefore protection against an excessive effect of thionamides.
2. During treatment with thionamides, little thyroid hormone is formed. The body senses a deficiency of the hormone. As a counterregulation, TSH is released from the pituitary gland and the thyroid gland enlarges. This can cause considerable problems (see section "What Is the Task of the Thyroid Gland?").

In rare cases—because of ineffectiveness, ADRs, or interactions—standard treatment of hyperthyroidism with thionamides plus a small amount of thyroid hormone cannot be used. In these cases, the thyroid gland can be destroyed with radioactive iodine.

How Do I Know I Have Hypothyroidism?

The leading symptoms of hypothyroidism are opposite to the symptoms of hyperthyroidism: a patient with hypothyroidism complains of dizziness, fatigue, sensitivity to cold, dry skin, constipation, and weight gain. In addition, hoarseness and hair loss can be observed. On physical examination, the doctor often finds a decreased heart rate, low blood pressure, and puffiness of the eyelids (myxedema).

Hypothyroidism is a common disease. A frequent cause of hypothyroidism is inflammation of the thyroid gland (autoimmune thyroiditis [Hashimoto disease]). In this disease, antibodies are produced that act against the thyroid gland. This leads to gradual self-destruction of the thyroid gland, with subsequent hypofunction.

In iodine-deficient environments, hypothyroidism can be prevented if iodized table salt is used and marine fish is eaten regularly. Manifest hypothyroidism that is due to iodine deficiency can be treated with potassium iodide (100–200 micrograms [100–200 µg] per day).

Overtreatment of hyperthyroidism with thionamides can lead to hypothyroidism, as can irradiation with radioactive iodine.

How Is Hypothyroidism Treated?

The goal of hypothyroidism treatment is to eliminate all symptoms and restore normal body functions (euthyroidism). The therapeutic goal for hypothyroidism is therefore the same as that for hyperthyroidism, except that the goal is approached from the opposite side. Hypothyroidism can be treated with thyroid hormone. The prerequisites for the success of the therapy are to take the appropriate drugs regularly and to exactly adapt the hormone dose to the symptoms.

So far, we have used the term "thyroid hormone", but, in the context of treating hypothyroidism, we need to discuss this term in more detail. Thyroxine (T4) is the inactive precursor to the active thyroid hormone, thyronine (T3). In the body, T4 is converted into T3 as needed. For the treatment of thyroid diseases, synthetic thyroxine (levothyroxine, T4) is preferred because it remains in the body for longer than T3 and guarantees a more even effect. The patient feels better with T4 than with T3 and does not feel as if they are "riding a roller coaster".

The dose of T4 must be adjusted to the individual so that neither hyperthyroidism nor hypothyroidism occurs. The therapy is started gradually with low doses, and the dose is increased at weekly intervals until the symptoms improve. In women, the dose is usually 75–125 µg of T4 per day; in men, it is usually 125–200 µg per day. Tablets containing the appropriate T4 doses are available.

The first signs of successful therapy for hypothyroidism with T4 are weight loss, increased appetite, less fatigue, and increased blood pressure. Hoarseness and skin symptoms improve later. The TSH level in the blood, which is determined regularly to monitor the course of the disease, should be low. A low TSH level prevents the thyroid gland from growing and thus avoids the mechanical problems affecting the throat organs that otherwise would arise.

To ensure reliable absorption of T4 into the body, it is necessary to take the tablets in the morning at least half an hour before breakfast with a glass of water (not with coffee or juice). Although this procedure takes some getting used to, a routine will develop over time. Because of the slow onset and long-lasting effect of T4, it is not a problem if you forget to take the tablets once (e.g., because you are traveling).

In pregnancy and during therapy with proton pump inhibitors for peptic ulcer disease (PUD) and gastroesophageal reflux disease (GERD), T4 requirement is increased. In patients with diabetes, T4 increases insulin requirement (see Sect. 6.1). In patients with coronary heart disease (see Sect. 5.2), T4 must be dosed carefully because the risk of myocardial infarction is increased. Avoid concomitant use of T4 and iron salts to treat anemia; otherwise, there may be a reduction in the absorption of both drugs into the body and thus weakening of their effects. An interval of at least 4 hours between the individual doses is recommended.

Misuse of Thyroid Hormones

The effect of thyroid hormones on metabolism and the associated weight loss is often abused. This is especially the case in professions where a low body weight is desired (e.g., in dancers and models). Taking thyroid hormones for weight loss or muscle building is not medically indicated and is life threatening. Uncontrolled use of thyroid hormones can lead to a deadly "thyroid storm". No antidote for thyroid hormone poisoning is available!

Stay Away from "Natural" Thyroid Hormones

On the Internet, "natural" over-the-counter thyroid hormones for treatment of hypothyroidism are advertised, which contain different and often undetermined amounts of T3 and T4. The emphasis on "naturalness" is intended to suggest that "natural" thyroid hormones are more effective and better tolerated than chemically produced T4. However, there is no difference in their chemical structures. What matters is the exactness of the dose, which can be provided only by chemically manufactured thyroid hormones. "Natural" thyroid hormone supplements are dangerous and make it more difficult to treat hypothyroidism. Don't be fooled by advertisements for them.

6.3   Osteoporosis

Summary

Osteoporosis is caused by an imbalance between bone-resorbing cells and bone-building cells. The aims of treatment are to eliminate the imbalance between bone breakdown and bone formation, and to prevent bone fractures. The basis of therapy is adequate physical activity, sufficient intake of calcium and vitamin D, and avoidance of risk factors and drugs that promote osteoporosis. Bisphosphonates inhibit bone resorption and can be used for all forms of osteoporosis. Selective estrogen receptor modulators (SERMs) are used in postmenopausal osteoporosis. A newer therapeutic option for osteoporosis and bone destruction due to cancer is use of antibodies that inhibit bone-resorbing cells.

Memo

- An active lifestyle is the best prophylaxis against osteoporosis.
- Vitamin D and calcium are the basis of osteoporosis prophylaxis and therapy.
- Bisphosphonates inhibit bone resorption in all forms of osteoporosis.
- Bisphosphonates must be taken with water on an empty stomach.
- Bisphosphonates can cause esophageal burns.
- Bisphosphonates can cause jaw damage.
- Prior to bisphosphonate therapy, dental restoration must be carried out.
- SERMs are suitable for use in postmenopausal osteoporosis.
- SERMs reduce the risk of breast cancer but increase the risk of thrombosis.
- Long-term oral therapy with high doses of glucocorticoids ("cortisone") increases the risk of osteoporosis.

How Does Osteoporosis Develop?

The human skeleton is not a rigid framework; rather, it is an active organ system and constantly adapts to physical activity or a lack thereof (e.g., due to confinement to bed or an inactive lifestyle). For the skeleton (as for every organ), the rule is "Use it or lose it!" In other words, the best way to prevent osteoporosis is to engage in regular physical activity that is adapted to the strength of the muscles and the cardiovascular system (see Sects. 5.1–5.3).

Bone-building cells (osteoblasts) and bone-resorbing cells (osteoclasts) are in balance in the healthy skeleton. If this balance between the two cell types is shifted in favor of the bone-resorbing cells, osteoporosis develops. Figure 6.3 shows this imbalance between bone formation and bone resorption, which

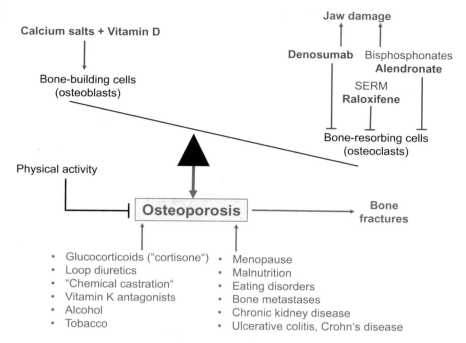

Fig. 6.3 How does osteoporosis develop, and how is it treated? In osteoporosis, the balance between bone-building cells and bone-degrading cells is shifted in favor of the latter. The basic treatment for osteoporosis is an adequate supply of calcium and vitamin D in the diet. With a healthy diet, expensive dietary supplements are unnecessary. Adequate physical activity is important. Most osteoporosis drugs are ultimately aimed at inhibiting the activity of the cells that break down bone. Different drugs are used, depending on the specific form of osteoporosis. Denosumab and bisphosphonates (the prototype drug is alendronate) can cause severe jaw damage. Therefore, it is imperative that teeth are restored prior to treatment with these drugs. Caries and periodontal disease favor jaw damage during treatment with denosumab and bisphosphonates. Several drug classes can promote development of osteoporosis when taken for prolonged periods. A prominent example is glucocorticoids (see Sect. 11.2)

leads to osteoporosis; the scale is tilted toward bone resorption. Table 6.3 gives an overview of the most important drug classes used for treatment of osteoporosis.

Osteoporosis is characterized by reduced bone density and thus an increased risk of poorly healing fractures. Bone density tests allow precise diagnosis.

The imbalance between bone formation and bone resorption is the starting point for osteoporosis therapy. It is aimed at strengthening bone-forming cells and weakening bone-resorbing cells.

Table 6.3 Overview of the most important drug classes used for treatment of osteoporosis

Drug class	Prototype drug	Mechanisms of actions	Indications	Important adverse drug reactions (ADRs) and interactions
Calcium salts	Calcium carbonate	Incorporation into bones with the help of vitamin D_3; thus, bone stability is improved	Very inexpensive and effective prophylaxis and basic treatment of osteoporosis; sufficient vitamin D_3 intake is important	More than 1000 mg (1 g) per day may lead to calcium excess; calcium salts can inhibit absorption of certain antibiotics (tetracyclines and fluoroquinolones); therefore, they should be taken at least 2 hours apart
Vitamin D	Vitamin D_3 (inactive precursor)	Conversion to active vitamin D_3 in the body; thus, increased activity of bone-building cells and increased incorporation of calcium into bones	Very inexpensive and effective prophylaxis and basic treatment of osteoporosis; sufficient calcium supply is important	More than 1000 international units (1000 IU) per day may lead to calcium excess
Bisphosphonates	Alen**dronate**	Inhibition of bone-resorbing cells	All forms of osteoporosis if prophylaxis and basic therapy are not sufficient	Avoid simultaneous intake with calcium salts, milk, and juices; take on an empty stomach with water, while in an upright position; risk of gastroesophageal reflux disease (GERD); ensure good dental hygiene; danger of jaw damage; dental restoration *before* treatment is mandatory

(*continued*)

Table 6.3 (continued)

Drug class	Prototype drug	Mechanisms of actions	Indications	Important adverse drug reactions (ADRs) and interactions
Selective estrogen receptor modulators (SERMs)	Ral**oxifene**	Inhibition of bone-resorbing cells	Postmenopausal osteoporosis when prophylaxis and basic therapy are not sufficient	Hot flashes, strokes, deep vein thrombosis
RANKL (receptor activator of nuclear factor kappa B ligand) inhibitor	Denosumab	Inhibition of bone-resorbing cells	Postmenopausal osteoporosis and osteoporosis in men, especially in patients with prostate cancer or chemical castration	Jaw damage (as with bisphosphonates), unusual forms of femur fractures, calcium depletion, cataracts, intestinal inflammation, allergic reactions at the injection site

Drug-specific word stems are shown in bold text. Basic therapy with vitamin D and calcium salts is unnecessary if you eat a healthy diet. The key to preventing osteoporosis is an active lifestyle. It is often forgotten that bisphosphonates can cause jaw damage. Therefore, take bisphosphonates only after consulting your dentist. Bisphosphonates can cause GERD if not taken properly (see Sect. 3.1)

ADR adverse drug reaction, *g* grams, *GERD* gastroesophageal reflux disease, *IU* international units, *mg* milligrams, *RANKL* receptor activator of nuclear factor kappa B ligand, *SERM* selective estrogen receptor modulator

Sufficient exposure to sunlight and regular intake of vitamin D and calcium promote bone formation and thus counteract development of osteoporosis.

Diseases and Drugs That Can Lead to Osteoporosis

Malnutrition, eating disorders, gastrointestinal diseases (such as Crohn's disease and ulcerative colitis; see Sect. 11.2), and chronic kidney failure promote development of osteoporosis. High alcohol consumption and tobacco smoking are associated with increased risks of osteoporosis.

Some drugs increase the risk of osteoporosis. If osteoporosis is present, the issue of whether prescribing of such drugs is justified must be assessed carefully. Glucocorticoids (cortisone) increase the risk of osteoporosis if they are used systemically for long periods (see Sect. 11.2). Other drugs that promote osteoporosis include loop diuretics (see Sect. 5.3), cytostatics (see Sect. 11.1), inhibitors of female and male sex hormones, proton pump inhibitors (see Sect. 3.1), and certain anticoagulants (vitamin K antagonists; see Sect. 5.2).

What Is the Basic Treatment for Osteoporosis?

The basic aims of osteoporosis treatment are to supply the body with sufficient calcium to promote bone formation, and to inhibit calcium excretion from the body. These processes depend on active vitamin D_3 (calcitriol). Calcitriol is produced in the liver and kidneys from inactive vitamin D_3 (cholecalciferol), which is ingested in certain foods (e.g., fish) or is formed in the skin from a precursor molecule under ultraviolet (UV) radiation. Calcitriol promotes calcium absorption in the intestine and bone formation in bone-building cells, and it inhibits calcium excretion through the kidneys.

The basic therapy for osteoporosis consists of daily intake of 800–1000 IU of (inactive) vitamin D_3. Active vitamin D_3 manifests its optimum effect only if sufficient calcium is supplied. Calcium should preferably be ingested with food, especially in the forms of milk and other dairy products. People on a vegan diet must pay close attention to adequate calcium intake (e.g., by consuming mineral water containing calcium). If calcium intake from food is insufficient, calcium can be taken as a dietary supplement in an amount of up to 1000 mg (1 g) per day. If the limits for daily intake of vitamin D_3 or calcium are exceeded, the body may experience calcium excess. Calcium excess (hypercalcemia) can lead to kidney and urinary tract stones, nervousness, and heart palpitations (tachycardia).

Bisphosphonates

If basic treatment of osteoporosis with vitamin D_3 and calcium is not sufficient, additional treatment is required. Bisphosphonates are an important class of drugs used for this purpose. Their INNs can be recognized by the suffix "_dronate". Alendronate is a typical representative. Bisphosphonates accumulate in bone-resorbing cells and inhibit their function. They can be used in all forms of osteoporosis, including glucocorticoid-induced osteoporosis and bone metastases (see Sects. 11.1 and 11.2). Bisphosphonates are effective, especially in fractures of the femoral neck in postmenopausal women (see Sect. 7.1).

Bisphosphonates must not be taken together with calcium salts, juice, or milk. Calcium salts should be taken 2 hours after bisphosphonates; otherwise, there will be mutual inhibition of their absorption into the body (see Sect. 1.5). Bisphosphonates must be taken in the morning on an empty stomach, at least half an hour before breakfast, in an upright position with a glass of water. Thereafter, the patient must not lie down again. If the rules for taking bisphosphonates are not followed, serious and painful burns may occur in the throat, esophagus, and stomach.

Especially in the jaw area, the body needs active bone-resorbing cells so that the jawbone and teeth can adapt to the constantly changing chewing load. Therefore, inhibition of bone-degrading cells in the jaw can have negative effects. Bisphosphonates can cause damage to the jawbone, bone loss, and ultimately tooth loss. Therapy with bisphosphonates (in the context of cancer therapy with cytostatics; see Sect. 11.1) may therefore be started only if the teeth have been restored beforehand. It is important that you maintain good dental hygiene and visit the dentist regularly.

Bisphosphonates should not be taken by people with chronic kidney failure, PUD, GERD, inability to sit upright, or calcium deficiency. They should also not be taken during pregnancy or lactation. Bisphosphonates increase the harmful effects of nonsteroidal anti-inflammatory drugs (NSAIDs) on the gastrointestinal tract (see Sects. 2.1 and 3.2). The risks of GERD and PUD are increased.

Selective Estrogen Receptor Modulators

Before menopause, a woman is protected against osteoporosis by the female sex hormone estrogen. Estrogen is produced in the ovaries. With aging, ovarian function becomes weaker, cessation of menstruation (menopause) being the most visible sign. After menopause, women have an increased risk of developing osteoporosis (see Sect. 7.1).

Estrogen receptors are found everywhere in the body; therefore, estrogen influences all body functions. In postmenopausal osteoporosis, however, estrogen receptors in the bones should be the only drug target because targeting of estrogen receptors in other organs can cause problems (see Sect. 7.1). This can be achieved with use of selective estrogen receptor modulators (SERMs), which act only on selected organs. The INNs of SERMs can be recognized by the suffix "_oxifene". Raloxifene is a prototypical SERM. It reduces the risk of bone fractures in postmenopausal osteoporosis. It lowers the risk of breast cancer. However, raloxifene increases the risks of stroke and blood vessel occlusion in the legs (deep vein thrombosis). Therefore, women with these conditions should not be treated with SERMs. Raloxifene can cause hot flashes and influenza-like symptoms.

Denosumab

Neither bisphosphonates nor SERMs are perfect drugs, and SERMs can be used only in women. Therefore, alternative drugs were sought that are better tolerated and can be used in both men and women.

The result of these efforts is the antibody denosumab. It inhibits the function of the cells that break down bone in women and men. Antibodies are proteins and cannot be administered by mouth (orally). Therefore, denosumab is injected under the skin (subcutaneously). Because denosumab is applied only every 6 months in osteoporosis, it is convenient for the patient. However, allergic reactions can occur, particularly at the injection site.

In women, denosumab can be used as an alternative to SERMs. Denosumab is particularly effective in men who have undergone chemical castration with male sex hormone inhibitors because of prostate cancer (see Sect. 11.1). Like bisphosphonates, denosumab can cause jawbone damage. In addition, unusual forms of femur fractures may occur. Rarely, cataracts and inflammation of the intestines (diverticulitis) are observed as ADRs. Adequate calcium intake must be ensured.

7

Drugs for Her and Him

Abstract This chapter is about drugs that are used either in women or in men. The first section of the chapter deals with the hormonal, physical, and psychological changes that occur in women during menopause. Menopause is a normal phase of life. Depending on the symptoms, individually tailored options for hormone replacement therapy are available. Erectile dysfunction in men has many causes, including high blood pressure, diabetes, and consumption of tobacco, alcohol, and cocaine. It is crucial to identify and eliminate the causes of erectile dysfunction. Phosphodiesterase type 5 inhibitors (such as sildenafil) increase blood flow to the penis, improving erections, but must not be combined with glycerol trinitrate, which is used for treatment of angina pectoris.

7.1 Hormone Replacement Therapy

Summary

During menopause (cessation of menstruation), production of the female sex hormones estrogen and progesterone decreases. Estrogen affects many bodily functions, while progesterone mainly affects the uterus. Menopause is a physiological process. About one-third of all women go through menopause without problems, while the remaining two-thirds experience symptoms. These can affect many organs. Depending on how severe the symptoms are and where they appear, hormone replacement therapy (HRT) with estrogen, possibly in combination with progesterone, may be considered. The decision for or against this therapy is made on an individual basis. A healthy diet, an active lifestyle, and abstinence from tobacco products are important.

Memo

- Menopause is a normal event, not a disease.
- Lack of estrogen can cause various complaints.
- Systemic treatment with estrogen is used for hot flashes, nervousness, and depression.
- Local treatment with estrogen is mainly used for complaints in the genital area and pelvic floor.
- Progesterone can support the effects of estrogen and create an "artificial" menstrual cycle.
- Estrogen may increase the risks of breast cancer and leg vein thrombosis, with subsequent pulmonary embolism.
- A healthy diet, an active lifestyle, and abstinence from tobacco products are important.
- There is a lack of evidence of the efficacy of herbal ("natural") drugs.
- HRT should be used for as short a time as possible.

The Female Sex Hormones Estrogen and Progesterone

The physical and psychological life of a woman is regulated by the two female sex hormones estrogen and progesterone. Estrogen and progesterone act through receptors that control cellular processes at the level of deoxyribonucleic acid (DNA). The effects of estrogen and progesterone take time (in the range of hours to days) to become apparent.

Estrogen is produced in the follicles (vesicles) of the ovaries. The estrogen level rises during the first phase of the female menstrual cycle and reaches its maximum at ovulation, before slowly falling. Progesterone is mainly produced in the corpus luteum (the remnant of the follicle after ovulation) during the second phase of the cycle after ovulation.

Estrogen promotes growth of the endometrium and mammary gland cells, and it prepares the woman's body for pregnancy. Progesterone transforms the endometrium so that a fertilized egg can be implanted, and it supports pregnancy.

While progesterone mainly affects the uterus, estrogen influences a variety of bodily functions. Table 7.1 shows an overview of important organs whose functions are supported by estrogen. Particularly important target organs of estrogen are the skin, hair, breasts, brain, heart/circulatory system, muscles, and bones.

Table 7.1 Overview of menopausal symptoms and treatment options

What do I need to know about?	These are the most important facts
Physical and psychological changes and complaints	*Skin:* wrinkling, dryness *Head hair:* thinning, graying *Body hair:* increase (e.g., lady's beard) *Brain:* nervousness, sleep disturbances, irritability, decreased performance and memory, depression, decreased interest in sexual activity (loss of libido) *Breasts:* sagging, loss of elasticity *Cardiovascular system:* palpitations, sweating, hot flashes, dizziness *Metabolism:* cholesterol increase, weight gain *Genital area:* vaginal dryness, pain during sexual intercourse *Pelvic floor:* muscle weakening, uterine prolapse, involuntary urination when abdominal pressure increases (e.g., during sneezing) *Bones:* bone loss; increased susceptibility to fractures due to osteoporosis *Muscles:* reduction in muscle mass and thus reduced physical performance
Available hormone replacement therapy (HRT) drugs	*Estrogen preparations:* tablets, patches, gels, nasal spray, and intramuscular injections for systemic treatment; vaginal suppositories and vaginal creams for local treatment *Estrogen/progesterone combinations:* tablets, patches for systemic treatment *Progesterone preparations:* tablets for systemic treatment (usually in combination with estrogen); mainly used for menstrual cycle regulation (it is an "artificial" cycle)
Indications for HRT	This is an individual decision that you should discuss with your doctor; the benefits and adverse drug reactions (ADRs) associated with HRT, as well as concomitant diseases, must be considered; if HRT is used, the lowest possible dose should be used for the shortest possible duration
Advantages of HRT	With systemic treatment, the aforementioned physical and psychological changes and complaints are improved; with local treatment in the genital area, the effect of estrogen is limited to the genital area and pelvic floor; the risk of colon cancer is reduced with systemic therapy
Disadvantages of HRT	Increased risks of breast cancer, leg vein occlusion (thrombosis) with subsequent pulmonary embolism, gallbladder inflammation
Absolute contraindications for HRT	Breast cancer with the presence (expression) of estrogen receptors on the cancer cells, known leg vein thrombosis, history of a heart attack or a stroke

(*continued*)

Table 7.1 (continued)

What do I need to know about?	These are the most important facts
Relative contraindications for HRT	Liver disease, high cholesterol, high blood pressure, condition after a heart attack or a stroke, benign uterine tumors (fibroids)
Alternatives to HRT	Herbal preparations have no proven benefit; for treatment of osteoporosis, bisphosphonates or raloxifene can be administered; for depression, antidepressants and mood stabilizers can be used; antihypertensives are used for high blood pressure; statins are used for high cholesterol
Lifestyle measures	Avoidance of obesity, tobacco products, and high-proof alcoholic beverages; healthy, balanced, calcium-rich, and vitamin-rich diet to prevent osteoporosis; general exercise; pelvic floor exercises

ADR adverse drug reaction, *HRT* hormone replacement therapy

Every woman knows that her physical and psychological status changes during the various stages of her cycle. This is a direct result of normal fluctuations in the levels of estrogen and progesterone in the body.

What Happens to Hormones During Menopause?

Around the age of 45 years, changes occur in a woman's body. The follicles in the ovaries can no longer produce as much estrogen as they used to, and the corpus luteum is no longer as active. The body tries to counteract these changes, but it doesn't work in the long run. As a result, the woman's fertility decreases. Many women notice that their menstrual cycle becomes shorter and menstrual bleeding weaker. The drop in estrogen levels influences the organs listed in Table 7.1. At some point, menstruation stops. This point is called menopause. The exact timing of menopause can be determined only retrospectively when no menstruation has occurred within 1 year. The timing of menopause differs geographically, 50 years being a typical age.

Menopause is a normal bodily process, which mostly does not need to be treated. About one-third of women go through menopause smoothly. The remaining two-thirds experience symptoms. It is not possible to predict how severe the complaints will be and which organs will be affected.

How to Treat Menopausal Symptoms

Table 7.1 summarizes the treatment options for menopausal symptoms. The commonly used term "hormone replacement therapy" suggests that during menopause, production of estrogen and progesterone ceases. However, this assumption is incorrect, because the body maintains basal production of estrogen and progesterone in the adrenal cortex and adipose tissue. Therefore, better terms are "hormone supplementation therapy" or "menopausal hormone therapy" (MHT).

Supplementation of the reduced estrogen and progesterone levels in menopausal women is optional. Unlike treatment for high blood pressure (see Sect. 5.1) or hypothyroidism (see Sect. 6.2), HRT is not an essential therapy. There must be good reasons for it to be used.

Before a woman decides for or against HRT in consultation with her doctor, a few aspects must be considered. A healthy lifestyle is crucial for a high quality of life during menopause. This includes avoidance of tobacco products (which can cause strokes, heart attacks [myocardial infarction; see Sect. 5.2], and cancer [see Sect. 11.1]) and avoidance of high-proof alcoholic drinks (which can cause liver disease and brain dysfunction).

A healthy, balanced diet with plenty of fruit, vegetables, and fiber, as well as dairy products and fish, is important. Dairy products contain calcium, and fish contains vitamin D. Moderate sun exposure is recommended, as this activates vitamin D. Calcium and vitamin D intake can help prevent osteoporosis (see Sect. 6.3). It is important to get enough exercise in an enjoyable way, whether it is gym exercise, running, walking, or cycling. Exercise not only strengthens muscles and the cardiovascular system but also helps to prevent osteoporosis. It is important to maintain normal body weight, as excess weight puts strain on joints and promotes osteoarthritis and cardiovascular diseases. Obesity restricts mobility and thus increases the hurdle to exercising.

Many women associate the term "hormones" with a harmful effect on the body and therefore seek supposedly more tolerable and gentler treatment methods. This "hormone phobia" is fueled by aggressive advertising for herbal preparations that promise a good and "natural" life without hormones. But hormones are natural.

Herbal preparations made from yams, hops, and black cohosh are popular among women with menopausal symptoms. Herbal preparations are available without a prescription and thus allow low-threshold therapy without medical consultation. There is a lack of scientific proof of the effectiveness of herbal drugs for menopausal symptoms. It is often unclear which active ingredients in what quantities are contained therein.

Another major reason for the fear of HRT is that the results of an important clinical study on hormone replacement (the Women's Health Initiative Study) were interpreted in a biased manner. The headlines read, "Hormones increase breast cancer risk!" and "Hormones are dangerous!" However, it was omitted that increased body weight, smoking, alcohol consumption, and lack of exercise are far more dangerous than HRT.

Discomfort in the genital and pelvic areas can be treated locally with estrogen without it causing systemic adverse drug reactions (ADRs) such as an increased risk of breast cancer. This is because estrogen is rapidly broken down in the liver (see Sect. 1.5). Problems with the pelvic floor, such as involuntary urination during sneezing, can be treated with pelvic floor exercises.

In the case of symptoms such as hot flashes, sweating, mood swings, or depression, systemic treatment with estrogen should be considered. Numerous dosage forms of estrogen are on the market, and a suitable preparation can be found for every woman. The goals of treatment are to find the minimum effective dose of estrogen and to initially schedule the therapy for a maximum period of 2 years. Estrogen can be combined with progesterone in a variety of ways to build an artificial cycle (with or without menstruation). This requires cooperation between a gynecologist and the patient to find an optimal treatment. It is important to remember that menopause is a dynamic phase of life to which one must adapt.

Before your doctor prescribes estrogen (possibly in combination with progesterone to maintain an artificial cycle), contraindications will be checked (see Table 7.1). If no contraindications exist, at least a short-term trial with estrogen (+ progesterone) is justified. Within such a trial period, you will recognize whether the HRT helps you or not and whether something must be changed.

No single drug gets all the complaints under control. But, by combining various measures and abstaining from risky behaviors (tobacco use and excessive alcohol consumption), most women can manage menopause well. Unlike herbal preparations, estrogen and progesterone preparations with precisely defined active ingredients are a well-founded component of this treatment concept.

Consider Selective Estrogen Receptor Modulators, Statins, and Antihypertensives

In cases of severe osteoporosis, therapy with a selective estrogen receptor modulator (SERM) is initiated (see Sect. 6.3). The prototype drug is raloxifene. Raloxifene acts on the bones in the same way as estrogen (as an agonist; see

Sect. 1.4), but it inhibits the effects of estrogen on the mammary glands and uterus (as an antagonist; see Sect. 1.4). This may reduce the risks of cancer in these organs. However, raloxifene promotes hot flashes and vascular occlusion (thrombosis of the leg veins, strokes, and heart attacks; see Sect. 5.2). Hence, this drug is not suitable for treating systemic menopausal symptoms. High blood pressure is treated with the antihypertensives discussed in Sect. 5.1. Statins are used if the low-density lipoprotein (LDL) cholesterol level is too high (see Sect. 5.2).

7.2   Erectile Dysfunction

Summary

Erectile dysfunction (ED) is a common and distressing condition for men. It is caused by high blood pressure, diabetes, and consumption of alcohol and tobacco. Phosphodiesterase type 5 (PDE5) inhibitors are used to treat erectile dysfunction. They increase the flow of blood into the penis, thereby enhancing erection. ADRs result from vasodilation. Reddening of the skin, a drop in blood pressure, and nasal congestion may occur. PDE5 inhibitors and the drug glycerol trinitrate, which is used to treat angina pectoris, must never be taken together, because a life-threatening drop in blood pressure could occur. In overdose, PDE5 inhibitors cause blue vision.

Memo

- Erectile dysfunction often reflects vascular damage in high blood pressure and diabetes.
- Beta blockers and 5-alpha reductase inhibitors (5-ARIs) can worsen erectile dysfunction.
- Alcohol and tobacco consumption can cause erectile dysfunction.
- When used properly, PDE5 inhibitors are safe drugs for erectile dysfunction.
- PDE5 inhibitors can cause skin flushing, a drop in blood pressure, and nasal congestion.
- Combination of PDE5 inhibitors and glycerol trinitrate can be fatal.
- In overdose, PDE5 inhibitors can cause blue vision.
- Ineffective counterfeits of PDE5 inhibitors are common.

What Makes a Penis Erect?

Penile erection is a prerequisite for successful vaginal intercourse. Figure 7.1 shows normal erection, development and treatment of erectile dysfunction, and a dangerous drug interaction with PDE inhibitors. Sexual stimulation (e.g., touching, viewing images with sexual content, or imagination) releases the neurotransmitter nitric oxide (NO) into the nerve cells and the vascular lining (endothelial cells) of the penis. This activates an enzyme (guanylate cyclase) in the vascular smooth muscle cells that produces the intracellular

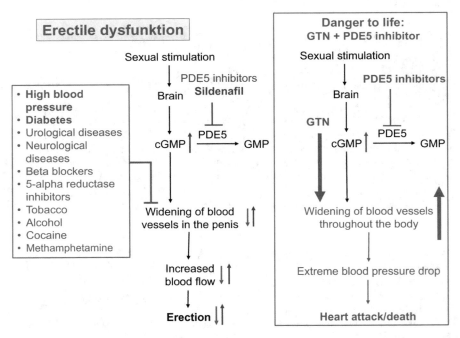

Fig. 7.1 How does erectile dysfunction develop, and how is it treated? (a) Cause and treatment of erectile dysfunction. (b) Dangerous drug interaction between phosphodi-esterase type 5 (PDE5) inhibitors and glycerol trinitrate (GTN). The maximum dose of sildenafil is 100 mg. It must not be exceeded; otherwise, "blue vision" may occur. For normal penile erection, the arterial vessels (blood supply) in the penis must be intact. The most common causes of erectile dysfunction are high blood pressure (see Sect. 5.1) and diabetes (see Sect. 6.1). It is therefore up to you to maintain your erectile function by treating underlying conditions. If you have angina pectoris (chest tightness with shortness of breath) during sexual intercourse, caused by coronary heart disease (CHD), *never* take glycerol trinitrate! It can cause a life-threatening drop in blood pressure, a heart attack, and death during sexual intercourse. First, have your CHD treated so you no longer experience shortness of breath. You can take a more passive role during intercourse

messenger cyclic guanosine monophosphate (cGMP). cGMP causes the arteries in the penis to dilate. As a result, more blood flows in and the penis swells. The swelling (erection) is increased by the fact that at the same time, the draining penile veins are pinched off and thus less blood flows out of the penis. After ejaculation (expulsion of sperm), the erection slowly subsides. This is due to constriction of the penile arteries (reduced blood inflow), as well as increased blood outflow through the veins. A permanent erection (priapism) is dangerous and can lead to death (necrosis) of penile tissue because the blood clogs the vessels (thrombosis). Therefore, it is important, on the one hand, that the erection works well, but also, on the other hand, that it does not last too long.

Two mechanisms ensure that in healthy men, a fine balance between stiffening and flaccidity of the penis is maintained and that priapism does not occur:

1. After sexual intercourse, less nitric oxide is released from nerve cells and endothelial cells.
2. cGMP is rapidly broken down by a special enzyme, PDE5.

After a time, which varies (the refractory period), another erection can occur. It is a common misconception among men that a particularly long-lasting erection is "good". On the contrary, the risk of priapism increases. Flaccidity therefore protects penile function. Erection of the clitoris in women works in the same way as penile erection does in men. The differences between men and women are not so big; it is just that in men, the erection is more visible.

How Does Erectile Dysfunction Occur?

Erection and flaccidity of the penis can be affected by a variety of factors. If a man suffers from high blood pressure or diabetes, long-term damage to endothelial cells in blood vessels can occur. This disrupts formation of cGMP and consequently impedes erection. It is therefore in every man's best interests to receive treatment for high blood pressure (see Sect. 5.1) or diabetes (see Sect. 6.1). However, men are less likely to go to the doctor than women. Men often do not see a urologist until they have erectile dysfunction. In many cases, a man does this not of his own accord but on the initiative of his partner. Such delays in seeking treatment must be avoided. Treatment of high blood pressure and diabetes is the best way to prevent erectile dysfunction.

Erectile dysfunction can occur in the context of neurological diseases. The most important example is multiple sclerosis, which affects younger men. Erectile dysfunction can develop after urological surgery, especially surgery on the prostate gland. The cause is usually nerve damage.

Certain drugs can cause or worsen erectile dysfunction. These include beta blockers (drug class B; the prototype drug is metoprolol), which are used in treatment of high blood pressure (see Sect. 5.1). Erectile dysfunction caused by use of a beta blocker is not permanent and ceases with its discontinuation. This ADR associated with beta blockers is due to vasoconstriction in the penis. Some patients notice the vasoconstrictor effect of beta blockers in their fingers (cold fingers in summer). If a patient with high blood pressure develops erectile dysfunction while being treated with a beta blocker, the drug should be discontinued and replaced by a drug from drug classes A, C, or D (see Sect. 5.1).

Another important class of drugs that can promote erectile dysfunction are 5-alpha-reductase inhibitors (5-ARIs; the prototype drug is finasteride). This drug class is used for male pattern baldness and benign enlargement of the prostate gland (benign prostatic hyperplasia). 5-ARIs cause reduced formation of the male sex hormone dihydrotestosterone, which counteracts head hair loss and leads to reduced growth of the prostate gland. Use of 5-ARIs in cases of baldness and benign prostatic hyperplasia must be carefully weighed up, because in many cases the ADRs caused by this drug class are irreversible after discontinuation of the therapy (postfinasteride syndrome). For benign prostatic hyperplasia, muscle-relaxing alpha-1 receptor antagonists (the prototype drug is tamsulosin) can be tried. In severe cases, surgical reduction of the prostate gland must be performed.

Consumption of alcoholic (especially high-proof) drinks and stimulant illicit drugs, such as cocaine and methamphetamine (crystal meth), may increase sexual desire (libido) in the short term, but long-term use of these drugs damages the finely balanced system of nerve, endothelial, and smooth muscle cells; thus, erectile dysfunction can develop. This is also true of tobacco product use.

Treatment of Erectile Dysfunction with Sildenafil

Sildenafil was originally developed as a drug for treatment of angina pectoris in coronary heart disease. However, in clinical trials (see Sect. 1.3), it was observed that many subjects experienced increased erectile function. Although development of sildenafil for treatment of coronary heart disease was discontinued because it was ineffective for that purpose, the drug was more successful for use in erectile dysfunction. This is a good example of how a "side effect" of a drug can become a "main effect" (repurposing; see Sect. 1.3).

Figure 7.1 shows how sildenafil works. Sildenafil inhibits the enzyme PDE5. As a result, cGMP is broken down more slowly, resulting in dilation of the penile arteries and greater inflow of blood into the penis. Sildenafil thus compensates for impaired function of nerve and endothelial cells. The drug has no effect without sexual stimulation; it does not cause spontaneous erection or priapism. Residual function of nitric oxide–forming nerve and endothelial cells must still be present. In severe cases of erectile dysfunction, sildenafil no longer has an effect, no matter how high the dose is.

PDE5 is present in large amounts in the smooth muscle cells of the penis. Hence, the PDE5 inhibitor sildenafil has a significant effect on an erection. The bladder contains PDE5 as well. Here, PDE5 inhibition leads to relaxation of the bladder and a reduction in the urge to urinate. This can be used in patients who have benign prostatic hyperplasia with an increased urge to urinate (pollakiuria). PDE5 inhibition leads to relaxation of the pulmonary arteries. This effect can be used in the case of narrowing of the pulmonary arteries (pulmonary artery stenosis).

PDE5 is present to a lesser extent in the skin, nasal mucosa, and gastric inlet. Relaxation of smooth muscle cells occurs in these organs. This manifests itself in reddening of the skin (especially on the face and upper body), a stuffy nose, and gastroesophageal reflux.

Phosphodiesterase type 6 (PDE6), which is related to PDE5, is present in the retina of the eye and is important for the normal process of vision. In high doses, sildenafil inhibits PDE6, which can lead to reversible visual disturbances. The patient sees their environment with a bluish tint. An important prerequisite for use of sildenafil is that the patient does not have any angina pectoris symptoms—in other words, that any presence of coronary heart disease is treated with the drugs described in Sect. 5.2.

Sildenafil is taken in doses of 25–100 mg about 30–60 minutes before sexual intercourse. Sildenafil works more quickly and reliably when taken on an empty stomach (see Sect. 1.5). The effect lasts for up to 3 hours. Sildenafil is suitable for planned sexual intercourse. PDE5 inhibitors with a longer duration of action (the prototype drug is tadalafil, which works for approximately 36 hours) are available. Sildenafil is available as a brand-name drug or as a generic drug. It is considered a lifestyle drug by health insurance companies for most patients and must therefore be paid for out of pocket.

Sildenafil interferes with physiological processes and therefore does not work only in patients with erectile dysfunction. This effect has contributed to the spread of sildenafil as a lifestyle drug. In healthy men, sildenafil causes erections with little sexual stimulation.

Sildenafil should never be purchased from obscure sources. Many of these preparations are counterfeits, which usually contain too little of the drug or no drug at all. In the best case, you are paying for an ineffective drug; in the worst case, taking too many of these "weaker" tablets can lead to unexpected overdose symptoms.

Nondrug options for erectile dysfunction include application of heat and use of massage oils or mechanical devices to increase blood inflow into the penis (vacuum pumps) or decrease blood outflow from it (penile rings). In the past, vasodilating prostaglandins were injected into the penis to increase blood flow and trigger an erection. However, this invasive and poorly controllable treatment method is strongly discouraged because of the risk of priapism.

Sexual Activity in Patients with Angina Pectoris

Sexual intercourse is associated with increased cardiac output, which can lead to angina attacks. You should have an exercise electrocardiogram (ECG) done before taking sildenafil if you have coronary heart disease. Alternatively, the patient may be advised to take a more passive role during sexual intercourse and let their partner take the initiative.

Simultaneous use of glycerol trinitrate for angina pectoris and sildenafil for erectile dysfunction is dangerous (see Fig. 7.1). Glycerol trinitrate releases nitric oxide and thus stimulates formation of cGMP throughout the body. As sildenafil inhibits degradation of cGMP, the whole body becomes flooded with cGMP. The result of this cGMP flood is massive dilation of blood vessels, causing blood pressure to drop sharply. In response, the heart beats faster and consumes more oxygen. This makes angina worse. Never try to induce a superhard erection by combining sildenafil and glycerol trinitrate. You could pay for this dangerous experiment with your life.

Caution with Methylphenidate and Antipsychotics

Sildenafil must not be used if you are taking drugs that can promote priapism. These include methylphenidate for treatment of attention deficit hyperactivity disorder (ADHD; see Sect. 9.1) or certain antipsychotics for treatment of schizophrenia (see Sect. 9.4). Sildenafil must not be used if you have ever had priapism. Sildenafil is contraindicated if you have significant curvature of the penis, because outflow of blood from the penis may be disrupted. Priapism can lead to vascular occlusion in the penis and loss of erectile function.

Sildenafil has been studied for its effect on orgasm in women. Sildenafil increases blood flow to the clitoris and vagina, making them wetter, but it does not increase the ability to reach orgasm. Sildenafil is not approved for use in female sexual dysfunction.

8

Drugs for Neurological Disorders

Abstract In this chapter, Parkinson's disease and epilepsies are discussed as prototypical neurological disorders. The first part of the chapter deals with Parkinson's disease, a neurodegenerative disease in which an imbalance between the neurotransmitters dopamine and acetylcholine develops. Accordingly, the aims of therapy are to strengthen dopamine and to weaken acetylcholine. With well-designed therapy, the quality of life can usually be maintained for many years, but Parkinson's disease cannot be cured. The second part of the chapter discusses epilepsies. In epilepsies, excessive nerve cell excitation occurs. Accordingly, the aim of antiepileptic drug therapy is to reduce nerve cell excitation. Specific antiepileptic drugs are available for treatment of different epilepsies and are also used for various other neurological and mental disorders. Antiepileptic drugs cause fatigue, balance problems, and dizziness.

8.1 Parkinson's Disease

Summary

Parkinson's disease is a neurodegenerative disorder in which the function of a specific brain region (the substantia nigra) is disturbed. This results in symptoms such as muscle stiffness, muscle tremors, and slow movement. In Parkinson's disease, the function of the neurotransmitter dopamine is weakened relative to that of the neurotransmitter acetylcholine. Parkinson's disease cannot be cured; only its symptoms can be alleviated. The aim of treatment is to strengthen dopamine and to weaken acetylcholine. By combining different drugs, it is often possible to enable good mobility in everyday life for many years. For each patient, a compromise between therapeutic effects and adverse drug reactions (ADRs) must be found.

Memo

- In Parkinson's disease, the effect of dopamine is weakened relative to that of acetylcholine.
- The aim of drug therapy for Parkinson's disease is to restore the balance between dopamine and acetylcholine.
- Dopamine precursors, dopamimetics, and inhibitors of dopamine degradation strengthen the dopaminergic system.
- Strengthening of the dopaminergic system improves impaired movement (akinesia).
- Strengthening of the dopaminergic system can cause nausea, vomiting, a drop in blood pressure, hallucinations, and addiction.
- Antipsychotics are dopamine receptor antagonists and can cause Parkinson's syndrome.
- Weakening of the cholinergic system with parasympatholytics improves muscle stiffness and tremors.
- Parasympatholytic can cause antimuscarinic syndrome.

Parkinson's Disease, a Neurodegenerative Disorder

All movements of our body require a finely tuned interaction of muscles. They are controlled by nerves that originate from the spinal cord. These nerves in turn are regulated by switching stations in the brain, such as the extrapyramidal system, which is regulated by the neurotransmitters dopamine and acetylcholine.

Parkinson's disease, like Alzheimer disease, is a neurodegenerative disorder. In Parkinson's disease, the substantia nigra, which is part of the extrapyramidal system, is progressively destroyed. Parkinson's disease occurs in older people (aged >50 years). These patients often have additional diseases and are sensitive to ADRs. Parkinson's disease cannot be cured. In most cases, the cause of Parkinson's disease remains unknown.

How Does Parkinson's Disease Develop?

Figure 8.1 shows the imbalance between dopamine and acetylcholine in favor of acetylcholine in Parkinson's disease, as well as the resulting clinical symptoms and targets for treatment. Table 8.1 summarizes the drug classes used for treatment of Parkinson's disease, which manifests in muscle stiffness (rigor), involuntary muscle trembling (tremors), and impairment of voluntary movement (akinesia). Muscle rigidity is recognized by a cogwheel-like resistance

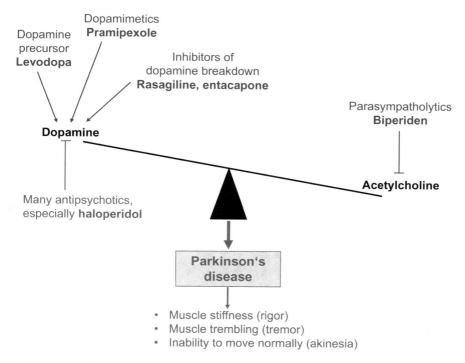

Fig. 8.1 How does Parkinson's disease develop, and how is it treated? Parkinson's disease is characterized by an imbalance between the two neurotransmitters dopamine and acetylcholine, to the disadvantage of dopamine. Accordingly, treatment strengthens dopamine and weakens acetylcholine. The available drugs can only alleviate symptoms. Drugs that boost dopamine improve akinesia. Drugs that weaken acetylcholine improve rigor and tremors. Antipsychotics (especially haloperidol in higher doses) can cause Parkinson's syndrome (see Sect. 9.4). This adverse drug reaction (ADR) can be prevented by a dose reduction or a switch to another drug

when the patient attempts to extend their flexed arm. Tremors result in illegible handwriting and difficulties in eating and drinking without spilling food or drink. Akinesia is recognized by a slow, shuffling, and small-stepped gait. Fine motor skills are impaired, and so is the ability to make rapid movements. Patients may initially notice difficulty playing an instrument or doing sports.

The brain can compensate for functional deficits. On the one hand, this is advantageous because it means that manifestation of Parkinson's disease is delayed. On the other hand, it means that the disease is diagnosed only when many nerve cells have been destroyed. Clinical symptoms do not become noticeable until approximately 70–80% of nerve cells in the substantia nigra are destroyed. This makes drug therapy more difficult. Drug therapy cannot stop the course of Parkinson's disease. The aim of treatment is to maintain as

Table 8.1 Overview of important drug classes used for treatment of Parkinson's disease

Drug class	Prototype drug	Mechanisms of action	Indications	Important adverse drug reactions (ADRs) and interactions
Dopamine precursors	Levodopa	Conversion to dopamine in the brain, replacing the missing dopamine	Parkinson's disease (this is the most important drug); mainly used to improve akinesia; almost always combined with the dopadecarboxylase inhibitor benserazide, which enhances the effect of levodopa by increasing the amount of levodopa reaching the brain	ADRs reduced by benserazide: nausea, vomiting, blood pressure drop: ADRs increased by benserazide: gambling addiction, sex addiction, shopping frenzy, hallucinations, confusion
Dopamimetics (dopamine receptor agonists)	Pramipexol	Agonism that acts on dopamine receptors, mimicking the effects of dopamine	Parkinson's disease: above all, at an advanced stage, conversion from levodopa to dopamine no longer works	Nausea, vomiting, blood pressure drop, gambling addiction, shopping frenzy, hallucinations, confusion
Inhibitors of dopamine degradation (catechol-O-methyltransferase [COMT] inhibitors)	**Entacapone**	Inhibition of the dopamine-degrading enzyme COMT, increasing the effect of levodopa	Parkinson's disease: add-on to levodopa + benserazide therapy if this combination is no longer sufficient	Nausea, vomiting, blood pressure drop, gambling addiction, shopping frenzy, hallucinations, confusion (but less than with levodopa + benserazide or pramipexol)
Inhibitors of dopamine degradation (monoamine oxidase-B [MAO-B] inhibitors)	**Rasagiline**	Inhibition of the dopamine-degrading enzyme COMT, increasing the effect of levodopa	Parkinson's disease: add-on to levodopa + benserazide therapy if this combination is no longer sufficient	Nausea, vomiting, blood pressure drop, gambling addiction, shopping frenzy, hallucinations, confusion (but less than with levodopa + benserazide or pramipexol)
Parasympatholytics (muscarinic receptor antagonists)	Biperiden	Antagonism acting on muscarinic receptors, counteracting the action of acetylcholine at these receptors	Parkinson's disease: add-on to levodopa + benserazide therapy, especially for treatment of muscle rigidity and muscle tremors	Antagonism at muscarinic receptors causes antimuscarinic syndrome (dry mouth; hot, dry skin; palpitations; blood pressure drop; constipation; urinary retention)

Drug-specific word stems are shown in bold text. Levodopa + benserazide, pramipexole, entacapone, and rasagiline mainly improve akinesia, while biperiden mainly improves rigor and tremors. The choice of drugs is made individually, depending on the predominant symptoms and their severity. The drugs have only symptomatic effects and cannot cure Parkinson's disease

ADR adverse drug reaction, *COMT* catechol-O-methyltransferase, *MAO-B* monoamine oxidase-B

high a quality of life as possible. Treatment of a patient with Parkinson's disease must be accompanied by physiotherapy to maintain mobility and dexterity. Physical rest and avoidance of movement are counterproductive in Parkinson's disease.

Parkinson's Syndrome Caused by Antipsychotics

Parkinson's syndrome can be triggered by various antipsychotics (Fig. 8.1) (see Sect. 9.4). In this case, the symptoms are not caused by degeneration of nerve cells. Many antipsychotics are antagonists at dopamine receptors and thus block the effects of dopamine. On the one hand, this is important for therapeutic effects in schizophrenia and bipolar disorder (see Sects. 9.3 and 9.4), but, on the other hand, it increases the risk of Parkinson's syndrome. Three options to treat antipsychotic-induced Parkinson's syndrome are available:

1. A reduction of the antipsychotic dosage
2. A switch to another antipsychotic with a lower risk of causing Parkinson's syndrome
3. Administration of a parasympatholytic (muscarinic receptor antagonist)

How Is Parkinson's Disease Treated?

Parkinson's disease can be treated by strengthening of dopamine or weakening of acetylcholine (Fig. 8.1). Strengthening of dopamine mainly improves akinesia; weakening of acetylcholine mainly affects rigor and tremors. In most patients, treatment focuses on strengthening of dopamine. Weakening of acetylcholine is mostly used as an add-on therapy.

The standard therapy for Parkinson's disease is the dopamine precursor levodopa, which is administered orally. Levodopa is actively taken up into the brain and converted to dopamine. However, this treatment works only at earlier stages of the disease when there are still enough nerve cells in the substantia nigra to perform conversion of levodopa to dopamine. At later stages of the disease, levodopa no longer works.

Conversion of levodopa to dopamine occurs outside the brain as well. This can result in ADRs such as nausea, vomiting, and a drop in blood pressure. In patients with Parkinson's disease, a drop in blood pressure is dangerous and can lead to serious falls with a risk of fractures because these patients cannot keep their balance well. Therefore, levodopa is combined with a dopadecarboxylase inhibitor (the prototype drug is benserazide). Benserazide prevents conversion of levodopa to dopamine outside the brain, thereby reducing nausea, vomiting, hypotension, and falls. Another advantage of combining levodopa with benserazide is that more levodopa can reach the brain, and so the symptoms of Parkinson's disease are relieved more effectively.

Risks of Too Much Dopamine

An increase of dopamine in the substantia nigra is important for normal movement, but an excess of dopamine in brain regions that do not lack dopamine can trigger confusion, hallucinations, or addiction (shopping, gambling, and sex addictions). These ADRs can be caused by levodopa. It is important that the doctor educates the patient about these ADRs and involves family members in the treatment. However, it is almost impossible to control online shopping, online gaming, and use of online pornography sites. A compromise between the desired effects and ADRs must be found. The fact that dopamine plays a role in triggering addictive behaviors may lead to misuse of levodopa.

Options When Levodopa Fails

As the disease progresses, more nerve cells are destroyed and conversion of levodopa to dopamine in the brain no longer works well. In these cases, it is possible to administer additional drugs that inhibit breakdown of dopamine and enhance the effect of levodopa. Inhibitors of catechol-O-methyltransferase (COMT; the prototype drug is entacapone) or inhibitors of monoamine oxidase-B (MAO-B; the prototype drug is rasagiline) are options. COMT inhibitors and MAO-B inhibitors are associated with the same ADRs as levodopa.

When levodopa and additional medications are no longer effective, dopamine receptor agonists (dopamimetics; the prototype drug is pramipexole) can be administered (see Sect. 1.5). Therapeutic effects can still be achieved with these drugs, but ultimately their effect diminishes. At the most severe stages of the disease, electrodes can be implanted in certain areas of the brain to improve symptoms.

Inhibition of Acetylcholine

Another therapeutic approach in Parkinson's disease is to weaken the function of acetylcholine. This can be done with parasympatholytics. These drugs are muscarinic receptor antagonists, neutralize the effects of acetylcholine at its receptors, and have beneficial effects particularly on muscle stiffness and tremors. Biperiden is the prototype of this class of drugs. However, the importance of muscarinic receptor antagonists in treatment of Parkinson's disease has declined. One reason for this is the limited therapeutic effect of these drugs. Another reason is that muscarinic receptor antagonists can trigger antimuscarinic (anticholinergic) syndrome, with a dry mouth; gastroesophageal reflux; hot, dry skin; palpitations; hypotension; urinary retention; and constipation. This syndrome can also occur with several other drug classes (e.g., nonselective monoamine reuptake inhibitors [NSMRIs]; see Sect. 9.2). In elderly patients, antimuscarinic syndrome is dangerous and often leads to admission to an emergency room.

8.2   Epilepsies

Summary

Epilepsies are characterized by excessive nerve cell excitation in the brain. The distinction between generalized and focal seizures depends on where this excitation occurs. To achieve freedom from seizures, antiepileptic drugs are used. They either block excitatory sodium or calcium channels or they enhance the effect of inhibitory neurotransmitters in the brain. Antiepileptic drugs can be used for various other neurological and mental disorders. Antiepileptic drugs can cause fatigue, dizziness, balance disorders, and double vision.

Memo

- Antiepileptic drugs are used for epilepsies, polyneuropathies, schizophrenia, bipolar disorder, anxiety disorders, personality disorders, and posttraumatic stress disorder.
- A balanced lifestyle is important for successful treatment of epilepsy.
- Antiepileptic drugs can cause fatigue, balance disorders, dizziness, and double vision.
- Several antiepileptic drugs can cause malformations in the embryo and fetus. Nevertheless, treatment is continued during pregnancy.
- To increase the safety of many antiepileptic drugs, therapeutic drug monitoring (TDM) is performed during their use.
- It is often necessary to test which antiepileptic drug works best for each individual patient.
- Benzodiazepines and Z-drugs can be used for sleep disorders.
- Benzodiazepines, Z-drugs, and pregabalin can cause addiction.

How Do Epilepsies Develop, and How Are They Treated?

Figure 8.2 shows the development of epilepsies and the possibilities for treatment. Table 8.2 provides an overview of the most important drug classes used for treatment of epilepsy (and other neurological and mental disorders). In epilepsies, the balance between nerve cell excitation and calming is disturbed. Overexcitation of nerve cells occurs. Generalized or focal seizures can develop. During an epileptic seizure, the patient can endanger themselves by falling and having accidents, especially in road traffic. They can put other people at risk. The goal of epilepsy treatment is to achieve freedom from seizures. The

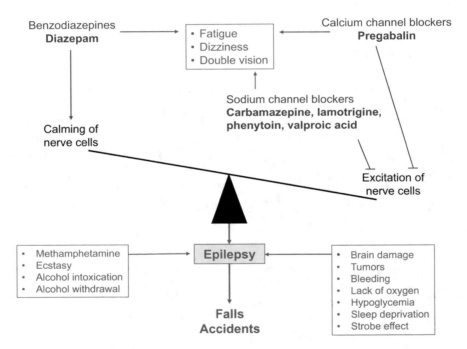

Fig. 8.2 How do epilepsies develop, and how are they treated? In epilepsies, an imbalance between excessive nerve cell excitation and diminished nerve cell calming develops. Antiepileptic drugs reduce nerve cell excitation and increase nerve cell calming. Drugs that reduce nerve cell excitation (calcium channel blockers and sodium channel blockers) are suitable for long-term treatment of epilepsies. Numerous drugs, overdoses of psychotropic drugs such as MDMA (3,4-methylenedioxy-methamphetamine, also known as ecstasy), and alcohol consumption can promote epilepsies. Many diseases can promote epileptic seizures. Hypoglycemia (low blood sugar) in patients with type 1 diabetes is a common cause of epilepsies (see Sect. 6.1). Antiepileptic drugs can be used to treat certain forms of pain (see Sect. 2.1) and various mental disorders (see Sects. 9.2 and 9.3)

Table 8.2 Overview of the most important drug classes used for treatment of epilepsies

Drug class	Prototype drug	Mechanisms of action	Indications	Important adverse drug reactions (ADRs) and interactions
Benzodiazepines: long-acting drugs	**Diazepam**	Enhancement of inhibitory effect of the neurotransmitter gamma-aminobutyric acid (GABA) in the brain; sedative, sleep-inducing, antiepileptic, antianxiety, and muscle relaxant effects; long duration of action (48–96 hours)	Emergency treatment for life-threatening seizures (status epilepticus); antianxiety and calming effects in depression and anxiety disorders; muscle relaxation for herniated discs; used only for short-term treatment, not for long-term treatment	Decreased alertness, decreased ability to drive, dependence and tolerance, unexpected agitation in children and elderly people, risk of falls, respiratory arrest when used in combination with alcohol or opioid analgesics, anterograde amnesia (sleepwalking, blackouts)
Benzodiazepines: short-acting drugs	**Midazolam**	Similar to those of diazepam, but with a much shorter duration of action (2–3 hours)	Difficulty in falling asleep, induction of anesthesia before surgical procedures, anxiety relief in myocardial infarction, status epilepticus; for emergencies, a nasal spray is available	Similar to those seen with diazepam; greater risk of anterograde amnesia with nasal spray (due to rapid brain flooding)
Calcium channel blockers	Pregabalin	Blockade of calcium channels, reducing nerve cell excitation	Neuropathic pain (e.g., in diabetes and shingles), anxiety disorders, add-on treatment for epilepsy; currently being tested for many neurological and mental disorders	Fatigue, dizziness, balance disorders, double vision, addiction

(continued)

Table 8.2 (continued)

Drug class	Prototype drug	Mechanisms of action	Indications	Important adverse drug reactions (ADRs) and interactions
Sodium channel blockers	Carbamazepine	Blockade of sodium channels, reducing nerve cell excitation	Many forms of epilepsy, bipolar disorder, schizophrenia, trigeminal neuralgia	Fatigue, dizziness, impaired balance, double vision, loss of effect with long-term therapy (due to accelerated degradation in the liver)
	Lamotrigine	Similar to that of carbamazepine	Localized (focal) seizures, add-on therapy for epilepsy, alternative to valproic acid in pregnancy (with a lower risk of causing embryo and fetus malformations), bipolar disorder (especially depressive episodes), migraine prophylaxis, schizophrenia	Fatigue, dizziness, impaired balance, double vision
	Phenytoin	Similar to that of carbamazepine	All forms of epilepsy (except for absence seizures), trigeminal neuralgia	Fatigue, dizziness, balance disorders, double vision, loss of efficacy with long-term therapy (due to accelerated degradation in the liver), increased body hair, gum growth
	Valproic acid	Similar to that of carbamazepine	Generalized seizures, bipolar disorder, schizophrenia, migraine prophylaxis	Fatigue, dizziness, balance disorders, double vision, particularly high risk of malformations (open back, open brain, neural tube defects) in the embryo and fetus during pregnancy

Drug class	Prototype drug	Mechanisms of action	Indications	Important adverse drug reactions (ADRs) and interactions
Z-drugs	**Zol**pidem	Enhancement of the inhibitory effect of the neurotransmitter GABA in the brain; weaker effect than those of benzodiazepines; mainly sleep-inducing and sedative effects; no antianxiety, muscle relaxant, or antiepileptic effects; short duration of action (1.5–2.5 hours)	Mild difficulty in falling asleep; used only for short-term treatment, not for long-term treatment	Fatigue, impaired driving ability, sleepwalking (anterograde amnesia)

Drug-specific word stems are shown in bold text. Pregabalin, carbamazepine, lamotrigine, phenytoin, and valproic acid are important drugs used for epilepsy. Diazepam and midazolam have many uses. Zolpidem is used primarily for difficulty in falling asleep. Pregabalin, carbamazepine, lamotrigine, phenytoin, and valproic acid are used in epilepsy and many other neurological and mental disorders. The effects of all drugs listed here are enhanced by consumption of alcoholic beverages, which must therefore be avoided

ADR adverse drug reaction, *GABA* gamma-aminobutyric acid

first step is to identify and eliminate the causes. If these measures do not suffice, antiepileptic drugs are used.

Epilepsies can be caused by brain damage such as tumors, bleeding (especially in the case of a stroke; see Sect. 5.2), lack of oxygen (e.g., in the case of heart failure), and hypoglycemia, especially in physically active patients with type 1 diabetes (see Sect. 6.1). It is therefore important that every patient with diabetes carries glucose with them so that hypoglycemia can be treated immediately. Lack of sleep and viewing of light flashes (a strobe effect) can cause epilepsies.

Drug abuse can promote epilepsy. Drugs that cause a massive release of serotonin in the brain (serotonin syndrome; see Sect. 9.2) are particularly dangerous. The psychotropic drug ecstasy (MDMA [3,4-methylenedioxymethamphetamine], which is very often abused as a mood enhancer at parties) is the most commonly implicated drug. Overdose of methamphetamine (crystal meth) can cause epilepsy, as can alcohol intoxication or alcohol withdrawal.

Some drugs can cause seizures, especially in the event of an overdose or poisoning. These include parasympatholytic drugs such as NSMRIs (see Sect. 9.2), scopolamine (used for motion sickness), biperiden (used for Parkinson's disease; see Sect. 8.1), and certain antipsychotics (used for schizophrenia or bipolar disorder; see Sect. 9.4). Theophylline, which is used in chronic obstructive pulmonary disease (COPD), may promote seizures (see Sect. 4.2). In these cases, careful consideration must be given to whether the drug can be discontinued or whether its dose can be reduced.

Mechanisms of Action of Antiepileptic Drugs

Use of antiepileptic drugs (anticonvulsants) is aimed at restoring the balance of nerve cell activity (i.e., exciting nerve cells less and calming them more). The first goal is achieved with calcium and sodium channel blockers; the second goal is achieved with benzodiazepines. Table 8.1 summarizes the properties of important antiepileptic drugs. The problem with all of these drugs is that they do not specifically act only on the neurons responsible for triggering epilepsy; rather, they act on all neurons. Therefore, antiepileptic drugs have certain ADRs in common. These include fatigue, dizziness, balance problems, and double vision. In many cases, ADRs must be accepted because freedom from seizures is of high priority.

Rules for Treatment with Antiepileptic Drugs

Several rules must be followed during treatment with antiepileptic drugs.

1. The drug dose must be escalated gradually to find the best balance between a reduction in seizure frequency and ADRs in each patient.
2. Therapeutic drug monitoring is important during use of antiepileptic drugs.
3. If a patient is seizure-free for 3 years, discontinuation of drug therapy can be attempted.
4. Because of possible interactions, use of any additional drugs must be kept to a minimum.
5. The patient must keep a seizure diary to monitor the success of the treatment.
6. Consumption of alcoholic beverages and sleeping pills must be avoided; otherwise, there may be an increased frequency of seizures and more severe ADRs.
7. Regular sleep times are important.
8. Antiepileptic treatment must not be discontinued during puberty or pregnancy, because the frequency of seizures may increase.
9. Kidney function, liver function, and blood cell counts must be checked regularly.

Use of Antiepileptic Drugs in Other Neurological and Mental Disorders

The term "antiepileptic drug" was coined to refer to drugs used for treatment of epilepsy. A patient with epilepsy understands that they are treated with an "antiepileptic drug".

For many years, there have been no drug treatments available for various neurological and mental disorders. These include trigeminal neuralgia, cluster headaches, migraines, polyneuropathies, fibromyalgia, schizophrenia, bipolar disorder, personality disorders, anxiety and obsessive–compulsive disorders, and posttraumatic stress disorder. Because of the lack of treatment options, doctors have tested antiepileptic drugs in such cases. Serendipitously, various antiepileptic drugs have shown good results in these "nonepileptic" disorders. Nowadays, use of antiepileptic drugs in many neurological and mental disorders is well established. This is a classic case of drug repurposing (see Sect. 1.3).

However, a major problem for doctors and pharmacists is explaining to patients why they need to take an antiepileptic drug for a disorder other than epilepsy. Dissociation between the indication and the drug class name leads to reduced adherence to treatment. To solve this problem, drugs should be named according to their mechanism. It will then be much easier to assign indications to a drug (see Sect. 1.3).

The broad efficacy of antiepileptic drugs allows important conclusions to be drawn regarding the origins of neurological and mental disorders. Our brain functions best when all nerve cells are in balance with each other. With overexcitation of nerve cells, an imbalance occurs and consequently a disease becomes apparent. Depending on which brain region is affected, this disease has specific clinical features, but the underlying mechanisms are the same for many diseases, and so are the drugs that are applied.

Carbamazepine, Lamotrigine, Phenytoin, and Valproic Acid

Sodium channels mediate influx of sodium into nerve cells and play an important role in nerve excitation. Accordingly, sodium channel blockers decrease nerve excitation. This effect is exploited in epilepsies and other neurological and mental disorders. Carbamazepine, lamotrigine, phenytoin, and valproic acid are sodium channel blockers.

Carbamazepine is used in various forms of epilepsy, bipolar disorder (see Sect. 9.3), schizophrenia (see Sect. 9.4), and trigeminal neuralgia. In the liver, it increases its own breakdown and also that of other drugs. For this reason, it is often necessary to increase the dose during long-term therapy and to watch out for interactions with other drugs (see Sect. 1.5).

Lamotrigine is frequently used because of its efficacy and tolerability. Unlike carbamazepine, it does not accelerate its own degradation. This makes long-term treatment easier. Lamotrigine is used for (particularly focal) epilepsies and bipolar disorder (especially during depressive phases; see Sect. 9.3), cluster headaches, migraine prophylaxis, polyneuropathies, personality disorders, and posttraumatic stress disorder. The drug can be dosed individually.

Phenytoin is effective in all forms of epilepsy except for absence seizures. It is used for trigeminal neuralgia. Like carbamazepine, phenytoin accelerates its own breakdown in the liver, and so the dose often must be increased in long-term treatment (see Sect. 1.5). Phenytoin may cause a cosmetically disturbing increase in body hair (hirsutism) in women by a mechanism that is not yet understood. This can cause significant problems in adherence to treatment and may necessitate a switch to another drug. Another problem with phenytoin is gingival hyperplasia, which not only is cosmetically disturbing but also can lead to tooth loss due to gum inflammation (periodontal disease). Therefore, it is imperative that patients treated with phenytoin adhere to good dental hygiene. If gum overgrowth occurs, it must be removed surgically.

Valproic acid is effective in generalized epileptic seizures, bipolar disorder (see Sect. 9.3), schizophrenia (see Sect. 9.4), and migraine prophylaxis. Of all antiepileptic drugs, valproic acid poses the greatest risk of causing malformations in the embryo and fetus. The neural tube is particularly affected. Nevertheless, antiepileptic treatment must never be stopped during pregnancy, because the risk of epileptic seizures increases during pregnancy and the embryo/fetus suffers serious damage due to a lack of oxygen during seizures. Therefore, pregnant women treated with antiepileptic drugs are monitored carefully during pregnancy. Neural tube defects can be diagnosed on ultrasonography. To prevent them, administration of folic acid is recommended.

Pregabalin

Pregabalin blocks calcium channels, which are important for nerve cell excitation. Pregabalin is popular as an add-on treatment when another antiepileptic drug is insufficient. The current focus of use of pregabalin is on polyneuropathies, which are characterized by burning and tingling sensations (see Sect. 2.1). Pregabalin is effective in diabetic polyneuropathy (a long-term complication of diabetes; see Sect. 6.1), and in polyneuropathy associated with shingles (see Sect. 11.3). Pregabalin is effective in anxiety disorders. It has considerable potential for abuse and addiction.

Benzodiazepines

Benzodiazepines enhance the effects of gamma-aminobutyric acid (GABA), the most important inhibitory neurotransmitter in the brain. Antiepileptic treatment is long-term. However, long-term use of benzodiazepines causes habituation and addiction. Therefore, benzodiazepines are used mainly in emergency treatment of life-threatening epileptic seizures (status epilepticus). Benzodiazepines are also used for short-term treatment of sleep and anxiety disorders (e.g., in the context of depression) and for acute back pain.

Many benzodiazepines are available. They differ in their durations of action. The international nonproprietary names (INNs) of long-acting benzodiazepines have the suffix "_zepam" (the prototype drug is diazepam), and the

INNs of the short-acting ones have the suffix "_zolam" (the prototype drug is midazolam).

Simultaneous intake of benzodiazepines and alcohol is dangerous. Benzodiazepines impair the ability to drive and the ability to operate machinery. Respiratory arrest may occur. In the event of respiratory arrest, an emergency doctor intravenously injects the antidote flumazenil, which rapidly reverses the effects of benzodiazepines. As a result of the muscle relaxant effect, impaired balance and severe falls may occur. When benzodiazepines are combined with opioid analgesics, the risk of falls is increased and respiratory arrest is possible (see Sect. 2.2). Benzodiazepines should not be used in children and the elderly, because in both age groups, these drugs often have paradoxical stimulatory effects.

Anterograde amnesia caused by benzodiazepines is dangerous. The patient does not remember events following the drug intake. During anterograde amnesia, the patient can walk around and cause accidents or become an accident victim themselves. The patient is unresponsive and, to other observers, they give the impression of being a sleepwalker. The risk of anterograde amnesia is high when the drug enters the brain rapidly (e.g., after being administered intravenously or as a nasal spray) and when it is combined with alcohol. Numerous cases of sexual abuse during this state have occurred. Anterograde amnesia is often mistaken for retrograde amnesia. In the latter, the memory gap exists for the period preceding an event (usually an accident with traumatic brain injury).

Z-Drugs

Z-drugs (prototype zolpidem) are related to benzodiazepines. They have mainly sedative and sleep-inducing effects. Z-drugs do not have anxiolytic, antiepileptic, or muscle relaxant effects. They are characterized by a short duration of action and are therefore mainly used for mild sleep disorders. As Z-drugs pose a lower risk of addiction than benzodiazepines, they are often prescribed too carelessly. The risk of anterograde amnesia with Z-drugs is underestimated, especially when they are taken in combination with alcohol (Table 8.2).

9

Drugs for Mental Disorders

Abstract Mental disorders strongly affect the quality of life, influence the family and professional environments, and are socially stigmatized and burdened with prejudice. Using the examples of attention deficit–hyperactivity disorder, depression, bipolar disorder, and schizophrenia, this chapter explains how mental disorders develop and how they are treated. Mental disorders are organic (they originate in the brain) and have psychological (mental) manifestations. The chapter explains which drugs should be taken for each particular disorder. It also discusses the adverse drug reactions associated with each drug. Cannabis products are linked to the onset of bipolar disorder and schizophrenia, and they should therefore be avoided.

9.1 Attention Deficit–Hyperactivity Disorder

Summary

Attention deficit–hyperactivity disorder (ADHD) starts in childhood or adolescence. In ADHD, a deficiency of the neurotransmitter dopamine is found in certain regions of the brain. The symptoms of ADHD are inattention, unruly behavior, and disturbed social relationships. Treatment of ADHD requires cooperation between the patient, parents, teachers, psychiatrist, and psychotherapist. Methylphenidate is the most important drug used for treatment of ADHD. It enhances the effects of dopamine by various mechanisms. Treatment breaks are important in methylphenidate therapy so that dopamine stores can be refilled. Due to its attention-enhancing effect, methylphenidate poses a considerable risk of abuse.

Memo

- Methylphenidate is the main drug used to treat ADHD.
- Methylphenidate enhances the effects of dopamine in the brain.
- Methylphenidate cannot cure ADHD; it can only relieve its symptoms.
- Breaks in treatment must be taken so that dopamine stores can be refilled.
- Methylphenidate has considerable potential for addiction.
- Methylphenidate works on people without ADHD and is misused for "brain doping".
- Methylphenidate suppresses the appetite and can cause sleep disturbances, high blood pressure, and permanent penile erections.
- Methylphenidate must be stored under lock and key.

How Does Attention Deficit–Hyperactivity Disorder Develop?

Figure 9.1 provides an overview of the development of ADHD and treatment options. ADHD is characterized by inattention; impulsive behavior; low frustration tolerance, low self-confidence; poor writing; relationship problems with parents, siblings, and friends; forgetfulness; and mood swings. Up to 3–10% of all children and adolescents suffer from ADHD. Boys are more frequently affected than girls.

Although ADHD is a childhood and adolescent disorder, up to 60% of all ADHD disorders persist into adulthood. The cause of ADHD is not known. As with most mental disorders (see Sects. 9.2–9.4), a combination of genetic factors and environmental influences contributes to ADHD. Imaging techniques have shown that a transporter (see Sect. 1.4), which sucks the neurotransmitter dopamine out of certain brain regions (in the frontostriatal system), is too active in ADHD. As a result, the brain is depleted of dopamine in this region. The lack of dopamine in ADHD is not the same as that in Parkinson's disease (see Sect. 8.1). ADHD is a neurodevelopmental disorder.

How Can Attention Deficit–Hyperactivity Disorder Be Treated?

An integral part of ADHD therapy is organization of everyday life. A clear daily structure is important. Overstimulation must be avoided. The times for dealing with electronic media (using smartphones, tablets, computers, and television) must be regulated. High-quality leisure activities (sports, playing

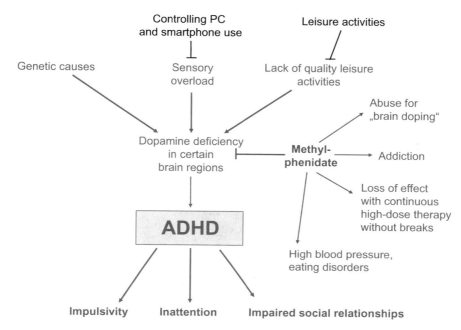

Fig. 9.1 How does attention deficit—hyperactivity disorder (ADHD) develop, and how is it treated? A dopamine deficiency in certain brain regions (in the frontostriatal system) plays an important role in development of ADHD. Unlike Parkinson's disease (see Sect. 8.1), ADHD is a neurodevelopmental disorder. Methylphenidate is just one component in the treatment concept for ADHD. Improper treatment with methylphenidate can cause significant problems. Therefore, access to methylphenidate must be strictly controlled. Don't ever try out "brain doping" with methylphenidate on yourself. Methylphenidate can cause addiction

an instrument, and outdoor activities) can improve ADHD symptoms. Successful ADHD therapy is possible only if there is good cooperation between the patient, parents, school, child and adolescent psychiatrist, and psychotherapist. This is a complex situation. Drug therapy is only one component of ADHD treatment.

Drug therapy is aimed at normalizing the function of the frontostriatal system and thus improving clinical symptoms. Methylphenidate (MPH) is the most important drug used for treatment of ADHD. Almost everyone knows the brand-name Ritalin®. As described in Sect. 1.2, brand-names should not be used in doctor–patient communication for various reasons; instead, the international nonproprietary names (INNs) of drugs should be used.

In the case of methylphenidate, however, the brand-name Ritalin® helps us to remember the important effects of this drug. The wife of the chemist who synthesized methylphenidate in 1944 was named Rita. At that time, clinical studies were not mandatory. It was quite common for scientists to test drugs by applying them to themselves or to family members (see Sect. 1.3), and so it went with methylphenidate. Rita, who was not an ADHD patient, found that methylphenidate made her a better tennis player. Therefore, Rita became addicted to methylphenidate, and her "self-trial" was "rewarded" with the brand-name Ritalin®. However, methylphenidate could not help Rita win Wimbledon. This anecdote summarizes four essential properties of methylphenidate:

1. Methylphenidate increases the ability to focus and perform.
2. Methylphenidate works in all people.
3. Methylphenidate has addiction potential.
4. Methylphenidate is not a wonder drug.

In recent years, the number of prescriptions of methylphenidate has increased substantially. Probably, many prescriptions are based on uncertain ADHD diagnoses and either the methylphenidate is then sold on the black market as a "neuroenhancer" or for brain doping, or it is consumed by healthy family members.

Methylphenidate mimics the effects of dopamine through dual mechanisms:

1. It enters nerve cells and causes the dopamine stored in them to be released. This mechanism is important in development of addiction because the release of dopamine is fast. In the section of this book that discusses opioid analgesics (see Sect. 2.2), it is mentioned that rapid uptake of drugs in the brain is an important factor in induction of addiction. This effect of methylphenidate depends on the presence of dopamine in the nerve cells; otherwise, no dopamine can be released. Without dopamine, methylphenidate is ineffective. The only way to replenish dopamine is to take a break from using methylphenidate and give the neurons time to refill their dopamine stores. As you can easily imagine, an ADHD patient does not feel well when methylphenidate stops working.
2. The second mechanism of methylphenidate is less dangerous: methylphenidate inhibits reuptake of dopamine into nerve cells. Dopamine is therefore available for longer as a neurotransmitter for nerve communication. In a comparable way, many antidepressants act on reuptake of serotonin and norepinephrine into nerve cells (see Sect. 9.2). This mechanism does not cause addiction.

The mechanisms of action of methylphenidate have important consequences for its use: it must never be taken without a break. In most cases, methylphenidate is not given over the weekend. During these treatment breaks, it is crucial that child and adolescent patients are offered good leisure activities so that their behavior does not escalate. It is dangerous to reintroduce methylphenidate too soon in the event of behavioral escalation or to increase the dose to "sedate" the children. Although there may be short-term success, the inevitable consequence of such a dose increase is that the dopamine stores are emptied faster; thus, methylphenidate no longer works.

Methylphenidate cannot cure ADHD, but it helps to integrate a child with ADHD into their environment. Methylphenidate is not a substitute for behavioral therapy. These measures complement each other. However, the treatability of ADHD by a drug can be a relief for the child, parents, and teachers because it demonstrates that the child's ADHD is an organic (neurochemical) disorder for which no one is "guilty".

When methylphenidate is administered orally, its calming and attention-enhancing effects begin after approximately 30–45 minutes and last for 3–6 hours. This duration of action is not long enough for many school days. For this reason, in various dosage forms available on the market, methylphenidate is released and absorbed into the body with a delay (see Sect. 1.5). The maximum effect is somewhat lesser, but the duration of action is longer. In addition, the risk of dependence is reduced by the slow delivery of the drug to the brain (see Sect. 2.2). Which form of administration and which dose are most suitable for each ADHD patient must be determined individually.

Methylphenidate Abuse

The attention-enhancing effect of methylphenidate in people without ADHD is well known and is therefore widely abused to improve performance in exams. Solutions prepared from capsules in "home laboratories" for intravenous use are dangerous because they produce a rapid flood of the drug into the brain (see Sect. 2.2). Methylphenidate triggers a vicious cycle in which the reward from the increase in performance leads to a further increase in the dose. However, the cycle does not last long. The dopamine stores in the brain are emptied quickly, and withdrawal symptoms occur. The abuser feels depressed and anxious, becomes aggressive, and comes into conflict with their social environment. They may experience palpitations, sweating, and trembling (see Sect. 2.2). Although these withdrawal symptoms can be alleviated by use of alpha-2 receptor agonists (the prototype drug is clonidine), they do not prevent the addicted person from having to go through a deep valley before their dopamine stores are replenished.

To prevent misuse of methylphenidate, it is important that parents store the capsules in a locked cabinet. However, there have been numerous cases of parents of ADHD patients making unauthorized use of methylphenidate to increase their own performance. The following measures help prevent misuse of methylphenidate:

1. The diagnosis of ADHD must be made by a psychiatrist.
2. The intake of methylphenidate by the ADHD patient must be closely controlled.
3. Society must be made aware of the risks of misuse of methylphenidate. This is the only way to prevent its misuse for unethical performance enhancement.

Methylphenidate acts predominantly on dopamine-releasing neurons and, to a certain extent, on norepinephrine-releasing neurons. This results in stimulation of the sympathetic nervous system, with palpitations and increased blood pressure (see Sect. 5.1). Therefore, blood pressure must be measured regularly in patients treated with methylphenidate. An increase in blood pressure indicates that the dose of methylphenidate is too high.

Activation of the sympathetic nervous system by methylphenidate leads to a loss of appetite and weight loss. In particular, young girls misuse this effect to reduce their body weight. Methylphenidate can cause a painful permanent penile erection (priapism; see Sect. 7.2). As this can lead to necrosis (death) of the penis in the worst case, methylphenidate must be discontinued.

9.2 Depression

Summary

Depression is a common mental disorder characterized by deficiency of the neurotransmitters norepinephrine and serotonin. Important connections between nerve cells are disrupted, and typical symptoms of depression develop. The sooner that treatment is started, the better the chances of success are. Several drug classes correct deficiencies of norepinephrine and serotonin. Use of antidepressants depends on the severity of the symptoms. Often the patient experiences adverse drug reactions (ADRs) at the start of treatment, and several weeks pass before the therapeutic effects manifest. During this intermediate phase, the risk of suicide is particularly high.

Memo

- Suicidality is a major danger with depression.
- Treatment of depression requires patience.
- The best results can be achieved by combining psychotherapy with drugs.
- The term "antidepressants" is misleading because these drugs are effective in many disorders.
- Overdosing of drugs used for treatment of depression can lead to severe poisoning.
- Antidepressants do not cause addiction.
- The doctor and patient must test which drug is most effective.
- In most cases, ADRs become less severe over time.
- When monoamine oxidase (MAO) inhibitors are used, consumption of wine and cheese can cause strong increases in blood pressure.

How Do I Know If I or Someone Else Is Suffering from Depression?

Depression is common. This disease affects the patient, their family, and their professional environment. Depression is one of the most frequent causes of incapacity for work and occupational disability. The sooner that depression is recognized, the greater the chances of successful treatment are.

The primary symptoms of depression are a depressed mood, lack of interest, and loss of motivation. Secondary symptoms are difficulties in focusing, low self-confidence, feelings of guilt, sleep disorders, loss of appetite, apathy (indifference), agitation, and suicidal thoughts. Depression is classified into different levels of severity. This is of importance for treatment. In mild depression, two primary symptoms and one or two secondary symptoms are present. Moderate depression is diagnosed if two primary symptoms plus two to four secondary symptoms are present. Major depression is diagnosed in the presence of three primary symptoms plus five or more secondary symptoms. Everyone should recognize the symptoms of depression because the sooner it is treated, the better the chances of success are.

How Does Depression Develop?

Figure 9.2 provides an overview of the development of depression and the various treatment options. Table 9.1 summarizes the most important drug classes used for treatment of depression. A combination of social,

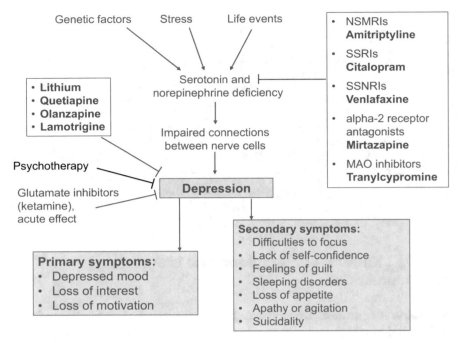

Fig. 9.2 How does depression develop, and how is it treated? Depression is caused by various factors that ultimately lead to deficiencies of serotonin and norepinephrine. Everyone should recognize the symptoms of depression. Besides psychotherapy, antidepressants (which address serotonin and norepinephrine deficiencies in different ways) are used. Lithium (see Sect. 9.3) and certain antipsychotics (see Sect. 9.4) are given in severe cases. A disadvantage of antidepressant drug therapy is that it takes several weeks for these drugs to show their full effects. The glutamate inhibitor ketamine is used for acute treatment of depression (see Sects. 2.1 and 11.1). It is often necessary to test different drugs and combine them with each other to achieve success

psychological, and genetic factors leads to deficiencies of the neurotransmitters norepinephrine and serotonin. These deficiencies are pronounced in the hippocampus, a brain region shaped like a seahorse. It is of importance to our emotional world, which is impaired in depression.

The amount and type of stress that people can tolerate vary from person to person. Therefore, one must not compare other people's stress with one's own stress scale. The term "burnout" is not a proper medical diagnosis but is often used as a more positive-sounding term for "depression". As a result of neurotransmitter deficiency, the connections (synapses) between neurons are reduced. Depression is an organic disease, just like a broken leg or appendicitis.

Table 9.1 Overview of the most important drug classes used for treatment of depression

Drug class	Prototype drug	Mechanisms of action	Indications	Important adverse drug reactions (ADRs) and interactions
Selective serotonin reuptake inhibitors (SSRIs)	Citalopram	Increased serotonin concentration in synaptic gaps (enhancing mood)	Moderate depression (level 1 of treatment), especially depressed mood	Nausea, vomiting, sleep disturbances, headaches, weight loss, decreased sexual desire, serotonin syndrome in overdosing or in combination with monoamine oxidase (MAO) inhibitors
Selective serotonin/norepinephrine reuptake inhibitors (SSNRIs)	Venlafaxine	Increased norepinephrine and serotonin concentrations in synaptic gaps (enhancing mood and increasing motivation)	Moderate to severe depression (level 2 of treatment): depressed mood and low motivation	Nausea, vomiting, sleep disturbances, headaches, weight loss, decreased sexual desire; in addition, palpitations, restlessness, and increased blood pressure; serotonin syndrome in intoxication or in combination with MAO inhibitors
Alpha-2 receptor antagonists	Mirtazapine	Increased norepinephrine concentration in synaptic gaps (increasing motivation in particular)	Moderate to severe depression (level 2 of treatment): low motivation	Palpitations, increased blood pressure, restlessness, loss of appetite (due to activation of the sympathetic nervous system)
Nonselective monoamine reuptake inhibitors (NSMRIs)	Amitriptyline	Increased serotonin and norepinephrine concentrations in synaptic gaps (enhancing mood and increasing motivation); in addition, a calming effect	Moderate to severe depression (level 3 of treatment), especially in agitation	Similar to those associated with SSNRIs; in addition, dry mouth, gastroesophageal reflux disease (GERD), and constipation (antimuscarinic syndrome); weight gain

(continued)

Table 9.1 (continued)

Drug class	Prototype drug	Mechanisms of action	Indications	Important adverse drug reactions (ADRs) and interactions
Monoamine oxidase (MAO) inhibitors	Tranylcypromine	Highly increased norepinephrine and serotonin concentrations in synaptic gaps (strongly enhancing mood and strongly increasing motivation)	Severe depression that does not respond to other drugs (level 4 of treatment)	Nausea, vomiting, sleep disturbances, headaches, weight loss, decreased sexual desire; in addition, heart palpitations, restlessness, and increased blood pressure; serotonin syndrome in combination with NSMRIs, SSRIs, and SSNRIs; life-threatening blood pressure crisis with consumption of tyramine-containing foods

Lithium is discussed in Sect. 9.3, antipsychotics in Sect. 9.4, and benzodiazepines in Sect. 8.2. The drugs listed here have different profiles and are used according to the symptoms that are present and their severity. For treatment of depression, SSRIs are the first choice, followed by SSNRIs or alpha-2 receptor antagonists, then NSMRIs and finally MAO inhibitors are used. Depression cannot be cured by "antidepressants", which are used not just for depression but also for many other neurological and mental disorders

ADR adverse drug reaction, *GERD* gastroesophageal reflux disease, *MAO* monoamine oxidase, *NSMRI* nonselective monoamine reuptake inhibitor, *SSNRI* selective serotonin/norepinephrine reuptake inhibitor, *SSRI* selective serotonin reuptake inhibitor

Who Diagnoses and Treats Depression?

If possible, depression should be diagnosed and treated by a psychiatrist. However, sometimes it can take a long time before you can get an appointment with a psychiatrist. Your family doctor can provide at least initial treatment in milder cases. Do not wait too long. Suicidal thoughts must be taken seriously. It is essential that you go to the emergency room. If you cannot go alone, have a relative or friend take you there. Your life is in danger!

How Is Depression Treated?

The goal of treating depression is to correct the neurotransmitter deficiency and to restore the connections between nerve cells. This takes time, from weeks to months. Figure 9.2 shows different therapeutic approaches to depression. In many cases, a process of trial and error is required before the right therapy is found. This poses a problem in that many antidepressants cause ADRs at the start of treatment, whereas a therapeutic effect takes weeks to achieve. Especially during this time, the patient needs strong emotional support from their doctor and their family.

Drug therapy should certainly be used in the case of moderate depression. Especially in the period between the start of drug therapy and the onset of its effect, suicidal tendencies can occur. So, keep a close eye on yourself during this time. If you are a relative of a depressed patient, you must take suicidal intentions or actions seriously during the transitional period, and take the patient to a doctor immediately.

How can this transitional phase be bridged? First, the patient can be prescribed anxiety-relieving drugs from the benzodiazepine class (e.g., diazepam) for a few weeks. However, caution is needed because these drugs have addiction potential (see Sect. 8.2). In the event of an overdose, and especially when used in combination with alcohol, benzodiazepines can lead to respiratory arrest and death. Antidepressants, which enhance the effects of noradrenaline and serotonin, can cause severe poisoning in an overdose. One of the most important precautions in initial treatment of depression is never to prescribe large packs of benzodiazepines or antidepressants.

Ketamine

The problem of the delayed onset of action of antidepressants has led to development of new drugs for depression. The aim is to achieve antidepressant effects as quickly as possible. Ketamine is a glutamate inhibitor (see Sect. 2.1) and is used in emergency medicine, anesthesia, and oncology for treatment of pain (see Sect. 11.1). Ketamine produces rapid-onset antidepressant effects in patients with severe depression but has addiction potential.

Antidepressants Have Many Uses

Many drugs used for treatment of depression enhance the effects of norepinephrine and serotonin. Originally, these drugs were developed for use in depression. For this reason, they are classified as antidepressants. However, these drugs are also used to treat other mental or neurological disorders. These include anxiety disorders, obsessive–compulsive disorders, posttraumatic stress disorder, and chronic pain. Because the use of norepinephrine- and serotonin-enhancing drugs has expanded and the term "antidepressants" continues to be stigmatizing, this term should be replaced by the more accurate term "norepinephrine- and serotonin-enhancing drugs". Norepinephrine- and serotonin-enhancing drugs are used for various mental disorders and chronic pain (see Sect. 2.1).

Are Antidepressants Ineffective?

It is often claimed that antidepressants are ineffective. A follow-up analysis of many studies (known as a meta-analysis) has shown that the therapeutic success of antidepressants is mainly (about 60–70%) due to their pharmacological effect, while the placebo effect (see Sect. 1.1) accounts for about 30–40% of their success. Antidepressants are not wonder drugs, but they are not ineffective either. The effect is dependent on the individual patient.

Do Antidepressants Cause Addiction?

Many patients are afraid of becoming addicted to antidepressants. However, norepinephrine- and serotonin-enhancing drugs work differently from benzodiazepines and opioid analgesics, which can cause addiction (see Sects. 2.2 and 8.2). Norepinephrine- and serotonin-enhancing drugs do not cause addiction. Discontinuation of antidepressant treatment must be done gradually; otherwise, unpleasant disease symptoms can occur, which are often mistaken for symptoms of withdrawal from addictive drugs.

How to Choose an Antidepressant

The choice of an antidepressant is made individually, depending on which symptoms are dominant. If the patient's primary symptom is loss of motivation, a drug that increases norepinephrine is indicated. If a depressive mood is dominant, the aim is to increase serotonin. If a patient suffers from both symptoms (less motivation and a depressive mood), an increase in both neurotransmitters is necessary. Norepinephrine enhances motivation; serotonin enhances mood. Since antidepressant effects of drugs cannot be objectively assessed, your doctor relies on your feedback as to whether the drug helps you.

Norepinephrine and serotonin are important for the function of the hippocampus and many other bodily functions. Unfortunately, it is not possible to increase norepinephrine and serotonin only in the hippocampus. These neurotransmitters are increased everywhere in the body. Therefore, use of antidepressants can cause many ADRs (see Table 9.1). ADRs caused by norepinephrine- and serotonin-enhancing drugs usually become less severe with long-term therapy.

How to Start Treatment for Depression

Selective serotonin reuptake inhibitors (SSRIs) are often used at the start of treatment. These drugs, as the drug class name indicates, inhibit reuptake of serotonin into nerve cells. As a result, more serotonin is available for communication between nerve cells, which therefore improves.

Because serotonin plays a role in many bodily functions, SSRIs can cause many ADRs. These include nausea, vomiting, sleep disturbances, headaches, weight loss, and decreased libido (which is decreased in depression). The many ADRs associated with SSRIs are a problem especially at the start of treatment but usually subside later.

After 3–4 weeks, you can expect an antidepressant effect to become apparent. If no such effect occurs, an increase in the dose or a switch to another drug may be considered. SSRIs must never be discontinued abruptly. SSRIs can be used in children and adolescents, but this should be done with caution because the developing brain reacts differently from the adult brain. In some studies, increased suicidality has been observed in adolescents taking SSRIs.

Poisoning with SSRIs is dangerous. It occurs with suicidal intent in depressed patients or by accident in children. As antidepressants are often prescribed in bulk, it is essential that these drugs are kept under lock and key and are not accessible to children.

SSRI intoxication manifests itself as serotonin syndrome. The body is flooded with serotonin, causing an increase in blood pressure, a racing heart, nausea, vomiting and diarrhea, sweating, confusion, seizures, and delusions. Often, empty antidepressant packages provide a clue that serotonin syndrome is present. Serotonin syndrome is life threatening and requires intensive medical care.

How Is Depression Treated When Selective Serotonin Reuptake Inhibitors Do Not Work?

At the second stage of depression treatment, drugs that increase both serotonin and norepinephrine are often used. Venlafaxine is a prototypical selective serotonin/norepinephrine reuptake inhibitor (SSNRI). Venlafaxine is prescribed when a depressive mood is accompanied by lack of motivation. SSNRIs can cause ADRs that are due to increased serotonin and norepinephrine. Restlessness, palpitations, increased blood pressure, and loss of appetite are observed.

If depression is primarily characterized by a lack of motivation, alpha-2 receptor antagonists can be used. Mirtazapine is a prototypical drug of this class. It increases the effect of norepinephrine. Palpitations, high blood pressure, restlessness, and loss of appetite are the main ADRs.

What Can Be Done If This Therapy Doesn't Help Either?

If the drug classes discussed so far do not work, nonselective monoamine reuptake inhibitors (NSMRIs) are used. These drugs are also known as tricyclic antidepressants (TCAs) because they chemically consist of three ring systems.

NSMRIs have been on the market for many decades. Therefore, their therapeutic effects and the ADRs associated with them are well known. They have a stronger overall antidepressant effect than SSRIs and SSNRIs but can cause many ADRs. Like SSNRIs, NSMRIs inhibit reuptake of norepinephrine and serotonin into nerve cells, thereby increasing their concentrations.

The term "nonselective" indicates that these drugs have effects other than inhibition of norepinephrine and serotonin reuptake. Amitriptyline is a commonly prescribed NSMRI. It causes fatigue in low doses. This effect is due to antagonism at histamine H_1 receptors, as with first-generation antihistamines (see Sects. 1.4 and 4.1). It can be used therapeutically when the patient is agitated. In long-term therapy, like many antipsychotics (see Sect. 9.4), amitriptyline can cause weight gain due to H_1 receptor antagonism.

Two other undesired effects of NSMRI can occur. First, these drugs dilate blood vessels by antagonizing alpha-1 receptors (see Sect. 1.4), which can cause dizziness, palpitations, and a drop in blood pressure. Second, these drugs antagonize muscarinic receptors (see Sect. 1.4), which can lead to palpitations, a dry mouth, gastroesophageal reflux disease (GERD), and constipation. This antimuscarinic syndrome is caused by many drugs (see Sects. 4.1, 8.1, and 9.4). Amitriptyline must be dosed gradually to achieve a balance between the desired effects and ADRs.

What to Do If Nonselective Monoamine Reuptake Inhibitors Do Not Help

In some cases, the therapy outlined above is not successful. In such cases, lithium can be added (lithium augmentation). Lithium is mainly used in bipolar disorder and is therefore discussed further in Sect. 9.3 of this chapter. Prescribing of lithium is delicate and is reserved for psychiatrists.

Monoamine oxidase inhibitors (MAO inhibitors) are used in patients with severe depression. They inhibit breakdown of norepinephrine and serotonin to ineffective substances and thereby increase concentrations of these neurotransmitters. Tranylcypromine and moclobemide are representative MAO inhibitors.

MAO inhibitors must never be taken together with other norepinephrine- and serotonin-enhancing drugs; otherwise, massive increases in the concentrations of norepinephrine and serotonin may occur. The consequences are manifold and range from nausea, vomiting, and blood pressure crises to seizures. Treatment is symptomatic.

Avoid Chocolate, Cheese, and Red Wine if You Take Monoamine Oxidase Inhibitors

Taking MAO inhibitors can lead to interactions with red wine, cheese, nuts, chocolate, and bananas, which contain the biogenic amine tyramine. It releases small amounts of norepinephrine in the body for a short time, which is normally harmless. However, the situation is different in patients treated with an MAO inhibitor. In these patients, the norepinephrine released by tyramine is no longer broken down, and this can cause a hypertensive emergency (see Sect. 5.1). Patients treated with MAO inhibitors must not consume foods or drinks that contain tyramine.

Because of interactions with other antidepressants and with tyramine-containing foods and drinks, MAO inhibitors have had a reputation for being dangerous. However, when used cautiously and with due regard for their interactions, MAO inhibitors are effective drugs for seriously depressed patients.

Other Drugs for Severe Depression

As alternatives to the drugs discussed so far, certain antipsychotics (see Sects. 1.2, 9.3, and 9.4) can be used. They are antagonists at various receptors, which have quite different effects, including antidepressant effects. In depression, quetiapine and olanzapine are used. Treatment with these drugs is reserved for psychiatrists and is considered for patients with severe depression. The successful use of "antipsychotics" in depression highlights how misleading traditional drug class designations have become (see Sects. 1.2 and 9.4).

Ten Reasons for Taking an Antidepressant for Depression

Antidepressants do not enjoy the best reputation. There are ten reasons why a person suffering from depression should take antidepressants:

1. Antidepressants can improve your mood and motivation.
2. Antidepressants can be dosed individually.
3. Antidepressants can make your daily life easier.
4. Antidepressants can have a positive effect on your sleep.
5. Antidepressants can help you look positively into the future.
6. If your antidepressant is not working or you experience ADRs, alternatives are available.
7. Antidepressants can be combined with other drugs, such as lithium, if they do not work well enough on their own.
8. Antidepressants do not cause withdrawal symptoms.
9. Antidepressants do not cause addiction.
10. Antidepressants do not change your personality.

Herbal Remedies for Depression

Many people believe that "natural" drugs are better than "chemical" drugs. St. John's wort extracts are an example of a herbal drug offered in many forms in pharmacies and health stores, as well as on the Internet. St. John's wort contains hyperforin, which acts like an SSNRI. However, there are two problems. First, the exact quantity of hyperforin in many preparations is unknown; hence, hyperforin can be overdosed or underdosed. Second, St. John's wort extracts contain active substances that accelerate breakdown of other drugs in the liver; therefore, the effects of those other drugs may be reduced. Drugs whose effects may be impaired by St. John's wort include oral contraceptives (causing a risk of unwanted pregnancy) and drugs that prevent organ rejection after transplantation (see Sects. 1.5 and 11.2).

9.3   Bipolar Disorder

Summary

Bipolar disorder is characterized by mood swings that go far beyond the normal. Depressive phases alternate, often abruptly, with manic phases. Manic phases are particularly dangerous because they are often difficult to diagnose. In their course, serious financial and social damage often occurs. In depressive phases, the suicide risk is high. Lithium is the most effective drug for bipolar disorder. It stabilizes mood and reduces the suicide rate. Valproic acid is effective for mania, and lamotrigine is effective for depression. Antipsychotics and valproic acid are used for acute mania.

Memo

- The most effective drug for treating bipolar disorder is lithium.
- Lithium reduces suicidality.
- Lithium improves reintegration of patients with bipolar disorder into society.
- Lithium can cause many ADRs; therefore, therapeutic drug monitoring (TDM) is important.
- A low-sodium diet increases ADRs caused by lithium.
- Because of the suicide risk, patients with bipolar disorder should never be given bulk packages of drugs.
- Mood-stabilizing drugs do not cure bipolar disorder; they merely reduce symptoms.
- Valproic acid and lamotrigine are alternatives to lithium in certain patients.

How Does Bipolar Disorder Develop?

Bipolar disorder is characterized by excessive mood swings from mania to depression that go far beyond the normal (see Sect. 9.2). Depression can be diagnosed relatively easily, whereas mania is much more difficult to diagnose. This is because mania, especially when it is only mild (hypomania), is perceived as positive by the patient and by people around them. The patient is "in a good mood"; has positive charisma and good ideas; and is active, interactive, and creative. Many patients with bipolar disorder refuse to have their hypomania treated. However, the problem is that they often don't notice when the hypomania turns into full mania. Then patients can quickly find themselves in financial and social ruin.

The shift from depression to mania can occur within a short time (seconds). The commonly assumed sinusoidal curve with a smooth transition between the phases is in fact an exception. Abrupt mood swings make it difficult to deal with patients who have bipolar disorder.

In a fully developed manic phase, patients lack insight into the disease; they are often aggressive and blunt. They hardly sleep, talk incessantly, are agitated, and are often megalomaniac. Manic patients engage in high-risk financial transactions with disastrous outcomes. Often, bipolar disorder is not diagnosed until the patient has ruined themselves. Unfortunately, it is only then that patients can be convinced of their need for treatment.

Bipolar disorder is common. It affects 3–4% of the population at least once in their lifetime. Figure 9.3 shows the development of bipolar disorder and the treatment options. The cause of the disease is unknown. It is assumed that a combination of genetic and psychosocial factors disturbs the balance of neurotransmitters in the brain. Bipolar disorder can be promoted by hyperthyroidism, which is easily treatable (see Sect. 6.2).

An important factor in development of bipolar disorder is abuse of cocaine, methamphetamine (crystal meth), and cannabis products. It is unclear whether drug abuse contributes to bipolar disorder or merely triggers it.

Treatment of Bipolar Disorder

Since the cause of bipolar disorder is not known, it can be treated only symptomatically. In acute mania with aggression, hyperactivity, and delusions, the antipsychotics discussed in Sect. 9.4 provide rapid relief (often within minutes). Valproic acid, which is discussed in section "Treatment of Bipolar Disorder with Antiepileptic Drugs", is effective in acute mania. Lithium and

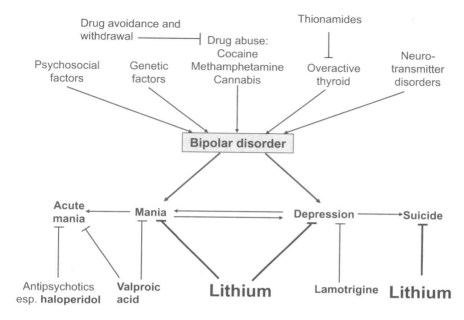

Fig. 9.3 How does bipolar disorder develop, and how is it treated? Bipolar disorder is characterized by abrupt and unpredictable changes between manic and depressive phases. In an acute manic phase characterized by delusions, antipsychotics such as haloperidol work well and quickly (see Sect. 9.4). However, the patient's lack of insight into the disorder is a major problem. Valproic acid (see Sect. 8.2) can be taken as an alternative to haloperidol. For mood stabilization in long-term treatment, lithium, valproic acid, or lamotrigine (see Sect. 8.2) are used, depending on the predominant symptoms. Lithium is the most effective mood-stabilizing drug and is the only drug that reduces suicidality. Although lithium treatment is effective, it must be well monitored because lithium causes numerous adverse drug reactions (ADRs). Abuse of supposedly harmless cannabis products can trigger bipolar disorder

lamotrigine have only a prophylactic effect. They are therefore called mood stabilizers and prevent or at least reduce the mood swings in bipolar disorder.

Lithium

The most valuable drug for bipolar disorder is the alkali metal lithium, which behaves similarly to sodium in the body. It is unknown why lithium is so effective in bipolar disorder. Like sodium, lithium distributes into every cell in the body. This explains why lithium can cause so many ADRs.

It takes about 2 weeks for lithium to develop its full therapeutic effect. Patients become gentle, sociable, and cooperative. The delayed onset of action must be communicated so that the patient, who is often agitated at the start of this treatment and lacks insight into their disorder, does not discontinue the treatment on the grounds of supposed ineffectiveness. It is therefore important to involve the patient's relatives and to convince them of the benefits of the therapy.

Why Patients Should Take Lithium for Bipolar Disorder

There are ten good reasons to take lithium in bipolar disorder:

1. Lithium has a reliable effect on manic and depressive phases.
2. Lithium is the only drug that reduces suicidality in bipolar disorder.
3. Lithium is usually well tolerated when therapeutic drug monitoring is performed.
4. When treated with lithium, the patient can communicate better with their family and social environment.
5. When treated with lithium, the patient is better able to pursue their professional activities and has less downtime.
6. Lithium therapy can be performed on an outpatient basis.
7. The patient is much less likely to require admission to a psychiatric hospital while on lithium.
8. When treated with lithium, the patient can manage their financial affairs much better.
9. Lithium improves the patient's insight into their disorder and cooperation with their doctor.
10. Lithium is not addictive and does not cause withdrawal symptoms upon discontinuation.

Adverse Drug Reactions Associated with Lithium

Lithium may cause tremors, slurred speech, confusion, seizures, palpitations, and a drop in blood pressure. Lithium causes thirst. As a result, fluid intake increases and the patient must urinate frequently. If the kidneys are not working well, water retention can develop, especially in the legs. Thyroid function may be affected and must be checked accordingly (see Sect. 6.2).

In the event of an overdose or accidental or deliberate poisoning with lithium, the ADRs described above are intensified. The diagnosis is confirmed by measurement of the lithium concentration in the blood. Lithium can be removed from the body by dialysis. To walk the tightrope between a good effect on bipolar disorder and ADRs, therapeutic drug monitoring must be performed during lithium treatment.

Lithium in Pregnancy

Since lithium is distributed throughout the body, it reaches the embryo or fetus in pregnant women. Lithium can cause malformations of various organs in the embryo and fetus, especially in the cardiovascular system. If a woman with bipolar disorder becomes pregnant, she should continue lithium therapy, because in pregnancy, bipolar disorder will worsen without therapy. Pregnancy must be monitored by ultrasonography to diagnose malformations in the fetus.

Caution with Nonsteroidal Anti-inflammatory Drugs and a Low-Sodium Diet

Treatment with lithium alone is usually manageable. However, it becomes more complicated if the patient must take additional drugs. Lithium should not be used in patients with severe heart failure (see Sect. 5.3) or kidney failure. If a patient with bipolar disorder is taking a nonsteroidal anti-inflammatory drug (NSAID), such as ibuprofen, for pain or inflammation (see Sect. 2.1), excretion of lithium from the body is reduced. In this case, the lithium dose must be reduced. If a patient with bipolar disorder is treated with a drug in class A because of high blood pressure, heart failure, or coronary heart disease (see Sects. 5.1–5.3), excretion of lithium is delayed. During concomitant use of these medications, the lithium dose must be reduced accordingly. It is widely assumed that a low-sodium diet is healthy and protective against high blood pressure (see Sect. 5.1). However, during lithium therapy, a low-sodium diet is dangerous because excretion of lithium is delayed and ADRs are increased.

Treatment of Bipolar Disorder with Antiepileptic Drugs

Lithium is the most effective drug for bipolar disorder. However, some patients cannot tolerate lithium or do not respond to it. For these patients, "antiepileptic" drugs are used (see Sect. 8.1). They inhibit disease-causing (pathological) nerve cell excitation, which is why they can be used in epilepsy. Since such pathological nerve cell excitations also occur in bipolar disorder, antiepileptic drugs have a mood-stabilizing effect. However, use of the terms "antiepileptic" and "mood stabilizer" for the same drug creates confusion and loss of confidence among patients and their families. This can lead to the drug not being taken regularly, because they may believe they have been given the "wrong diagnosis" or the "wrong drug". It is therefore much better to name drugs that are used in bipolar disorder on the basis of their mechanisms of action (see Sect. 1.3).

Valproic acid blocks sodium channels in nerve cells, thereby inhibiting disease-causing nerve cell excitation. This effect can be used in epilepsy and bipolar disorder. Valproic acid is effective in acute mania and prevents manic episodes. It does not cause addiction and does not cause withdrawal symptoms. For more details of valproic acid, see Sect. 8.1.

Lamotrigine blocks sodium channels in nerve cells. The drug is effective in epilepsies and prevents depressive phases in bipolar disorder. Lamotrigine does not cause addiction, and no withdrawal symptoms occur. For more details of lamotrigine, see Sect. 8.1.

The different profiles of lithium, valproic acid, and lamotrigine can be used to find the best possible mood-stabilizing drug for each patient with bipolar disorder. A switch to another of these drugs should be done with an overlap between them. Discontinuation of a drug must be gradual, so that a flare-up of bipolar disorder can be recognized and counteracted.

9.4   Schizophrenia

Summary

Schizophrenia impairs the ability to cope with everyday life, through the presence of positive symptoms (e.g., hearing voices) and negative symptoms (e.g., social withdrawal). Antipsychotics reduce the symptoms of schizophrenia and facilitate reintegration of patients into normal life. They do not cause addiction or withdrawal symptoms. Several antipsychotics are available and must be tried on an individual basis, depending on the patient's symptoms and ADRs. The most effective antipsychotic is clozapine. The disadvantage of clozapine is that it can cause depletion of white blood cells. Antipsychotics can cause cardiovascular problems, movement disorders, and weight gain.

Memo

- Antipsychotics are antagonists at many receptors for neurotransmitters in the brain.
- Antipsychotics act symptomatically in schizophrenia and other disorders.
- Antipsychotics do not cause addiction.
- Each antipsychotic is a drug with unique properties.
- Antipsychotics can cause cardiovascular problems, movement disorders, and weight gain.
- The most effective antipsychotic is clozapine.
- The blood count must be checked regularly during clozapine treatment.
- In dementia, antipsychotics should be avoided because they can cause severe ADRs.

What Is Schizophrenia?

Worldwide, about 1% of all people suffer from schizophrenia, and especially young adults are affected by this disease. The term "schizophrenia" comes from an ancient Greek term meaning "split mind". Unfortunately, that term does not capture the essence of the disorder; however, no consensus on a more appropriate name for this disease has emerged so far. Schizophrenia involves severe problems in all areas of thinking, feeling, and acting. Therefore, patients are unable to cope with the demands of life in their family, at work, with friends, and in society. Development of effective drugs for treatment of schizophrenia (antipsychotics) has enabled many patients with schizophrenia to participate, at least to some extent, in normal life.

Figure 9.4 shows the development of schizophrenia and its treatment. In schizophrenia, a distinction is made between positive and negative symptoms. This determines the choice of the drug. Positive symptoms, which are impressive and well known to the public—because they are often portrayed in magazines, books, and movies—include sensory illusions, hallucinations of an optical and/or acoustic nature (e.g., "hearing voices"), and delusions such as passivity phenomena (e.g., delusions of thought control by external forces). Less impressive, but more important for the prognosis, are the negative symptoms, such as social withdrawal, indifference, and lack of interest. Here, the transition to depression is fluent, which is reflected in the fact that similar drugs are used in these two conditions (see Sect. 9.2). Because of the combination of positive and negative symptoms, patients with schizophrenia often suffer accidents and social decline, with secondary diseases and a high suicide rate. Therefore, the average life expectancy in schizophrenia is shortened by

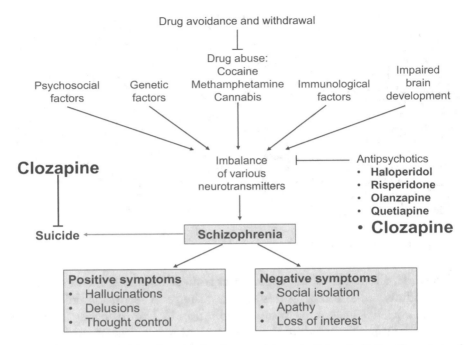

Fig. 9.4 How does schizophrenia develop, and how is it treated? Development of schizophrenia is favored by various factors. Abuse of supposedly harmless cannabis products can trigger schizophrenia. The disorder is characterized by increased function of many neurotransmitters. This leads to dramatic positive symptoms that are well known from depictions in books and movies. Less well known are the negative symptoms of schizophrenia, which show some overlap with those of depression (see Sect. 9.2). The aim of treatment is to inhibit the excessive functions of the various neurotransmitter systems with antipsychotics. Antipsychotics are antagonists at numerous receptors (see Sect. 1.4). The most effective antipsychotic is clozapine, but its use requires regular blood count checks because of the risk of white blood cell depletion. The traditional division into "typical" and "atypical" antipsychotics is problematic. Since it is not known exactly which neurotransmitter is disturbed in which patient, it is often necessary to test which antipsychotic works best in each patient

about 15 years. Drug therapy has a greater influence on positive symptoms than on negative symptoms. Clozapine is the most effective antipsychotic. It reduces the suicide rate and has a life-prolonging effect.

Crystal Meth and Cannabis as Triggers of Schizophrenia

As with depression (see Sect. 9.2) and bipolar disorder (see Sect. 9.3), the cause of schizophrenia is unknown. A combination of genetic and psychosocial factors favors its occurrence. Impaired brain development and certain immunological factors contribute to development of schizophrenia. Use of illicit drugs such as cocaine, methamphetamine, and cannabis products promote disease development.

Antipsychotics

Ultimately, all of these unfavorable influences lead to excessive function of neurotransmitters in the brain, causing the positive and negative symptoms. This model of disease development is supported by the fact that antipsychotics are antagonists at numerous neurotransmitter receptors (see Sect. 1.4). Clozapine is the most potent antipsychotic and, at the same time, it is an antagonist at more receptors than any other antipsychotic. Accordingly, broad-spectrum antagonism of receptors by antipsychotics is important for effective treatment of schizophrenia. This important aspect in turn contributes to better understanding of the disease.

Over 70 years ago, it was fortuitously discovered that the "antihistamine" promethazine exerted a calming effect in schizophrenia (see Sect. 4.1). This observation led to development of several drugs with the aim of finding the "perfect" antipsychotic. This goal has not been achieved, but antipsychotics with different profiles, different indications, and different ADR profiles are available. Therefore, in most cases, it is possible to find a suitable antipsychotic for each patient.

Ten Reasons for Taking Antipsychotics in Schizophrenia

It is important to convince patients that treating schizophrenia with antipsychotics makes a lot of sense:

1. Antipsychotics diminish hallucinations and delusions (including passivity phenomena).
2. Some antipsychotics (especially clozapine) act against social withdrawal, indifference, and lack of interest.
3. Antipsychotics allow many patients to live in the community rather than in psychiatric hospitals.
4. Depot preparations of some antipsychotics, ensuring a long-lasting effect, are available.
5. Many antipsychotics are available; thus, there is a good chance of finding a suitable drug for each patient.

6. Usually, a compromise between the antipsychotic effect and ADRs can be found.
7. Drug safety can be increased by therapeutic drug monitoring.
8. In the event of ineffectiveness or ADRs, another drug or combinations of different drug classes can be tested.
9. Antipsychotics do not cause addiction.
10. Antipsychotics do not cause withdrawal symptoms.

Antipsychotics for Emergency and Long-Term Therapy

In acute schizophrenia or mania (see Sect. 9.3), antipsychotics usually take between a few minutes and half an hour to have an effect (depending on the symptoms and the form of application of the drug) and thus allow rapid access to the patient. If positive symptoms dominate, treatment is usually started with haloperidol.

Schizophrenia requires long-term therapy. It is often possible to treat a patient with the same drug dose for many years. If a patient has problems in taking their tablets regularly, antipsychotics can be given as an intramuscular depot injection every 4–6 weeks.

Antipsychotics merely alleviate the symptoms of schizophrenia; they do not cure the disease. If an attempt to terminate therapy is made, it is important to taper off the drug. If treatment with an antipsychotic is not sufficient or is impossible because of ADRs, various other drug classes can be used in addition or alone. These include lithium (see Sect. 9.3) and antiepileptic drugs (sodium channel blockers and calcium channel blockers; see Sect. 8.2).

Typical and Atypical Antipsychotics

Table 9.2 summarizes the properties of five frequently used antipsychotics. The first highly effective antipsychotics (the prototype drug is haloperidol) were found to be effective against positive symptoms such as hallucinations and delusions (e.g., passivity phenomena). The antipsychotic effect of these drugs is mainly due to antagonism at dopamine receptors (see Sect. 1.4), which additionally play an important role in movement coordination in the brain (see Sect. 8.1). Therefore, these drugs may cause severe movement disorders (extrapyramidal symptoms [EPSs]):

Table 9.2 Overview of the most important drug classes used for treatment of schizophrenia

Drug class	Prototype drug	Mechanisms of actions	Indications	Important adverse drug reactions (ADRs) and interactions
Typical antipsychotics (mGPCR antagonists)	Haloperidol	Strong antipsychotic effect, especially on positive symptoms; changes in pain perception; no "sedative" effect; inhibitory effect on vomiting	Acute and chronic schizophrenia, acute bipolar disorder, chronic pain, severe vomiting; not used in agitation states in patients with dementia!	Dizziness, palpitations, falls, cardiac arrhythmias; highest risks (out of all antipsychotics listed here) of a wide variety of movement disorders
Atypical antipsychotics (mGPCR antagonists)	Clozapine	Strong antipsychotic effect on positive and negative symptoms, reduced suicide risk	Schizophrenia with strong negative symptoms, suicidality	Fatigue, dizziness, palpitations, antimuscarinic syndrome, low risk of movement disorders but high risk of weight gain, risk of white blood cell depletion (regular blood count checks required)
	Olanzapine	Antipsychotic effect, inhibitory effect on vomiting	Schizophrenia, bipolar disorder, compulsive disorders, vomiting with chemotherapy, severe depression	Fatigue, dizziness, palpitations, high risk of weight gain, risks of various movement disorders, low risk of white blood cell depletion
	Quetiapine	Antipsychotic effect, calming effect	Schizophrenia, bipolar disorder, compulsive disorders, anxiety disorders, Tourette syndrome	Fatigue, blood pressure drops, antimuscarinic syndrome, risks of various movement disorders, cardiac arrhythmias
	Risperidone	Antipsychotic effect, changes in pain perception	Schizophrenia, bipolar disorder, compulsive disorders, chronic pain, autism	Fatigue, dizziness, palpitations, risks of various movement disorders

Although the classification of antipsychotics into "typical" and "atypical" antipsychotics is problematic, it is used here for better orientation. Each antipsychotic drug possesses unique properties. Antipsychotics are used for many other neurological and mental disorders besides schizophrenia. All drugs listed here are antagonists at many neurotransmitter receptors and therefore have many uses and many ADRs. Clozapine is the most effective drug for schizophrenia, but it poses a risk of white blood cell depletion. Antipsychotics should be avoided in patients with dementia; otherwise, severe ADRs may occur
ADR adverse drug reaction, *mGPCR* multiple G-protein-coupled receptor

1. Initially, acute tic-like movement disorders of the face and neck may occur (acute dyskinesias). These are short-lived and can be treated with muscarinic receptor antagonists (the prototype drug is biperiden; see Sects. 3.1, 3.3, and 8.1).
2. Parkinson's syndrome (rigor, tremor, and akinesia) may develop between day 5 and day 30 of treatment (see Sect. 8.1) and can be reduced with biperiden, dose reduction, or drug switching.
3. After months, inability to sit still (akathisia) may occur, which manifests in patients walking around continuously. The treatment is the same as that for Parkinson's syndrome.
4. After months to years, chewing, lip smacking, and sucking (choreoathetosis) can occur. These ADRs are best treated by a switch to a different antipsychotic.

Drugs causing these symptoms are called "typical" antipsychotics. The aim was therefore to develop drugs with an antipsychotic effect but without the risk of causing movement disorders. As a result, the drugs clozapine, olanzapine, quetiapine, and risperidone (among others) were developed, and they are referred to as "atypical" antipsychotics.

The distinction between typical and atypical antipsychotics is firmly rooted in the literature, in medical language, and on the Internet, although this division is not accurate: with the exception of clozapine, all atypical antipsychotics can cause movement disorders. The term "atypical antipsychotics" is dangerous, because neither the doctor nor the patient expect movement disorders and therefore misjudge them.

"Antagonists at Many Receptors" Explains Therapeutic Effects and Adverse Drug Reactions

Because of the problems discussed above, the more accurate term "antagonists at multiple G-protein-coupled receptors" (mGPCR antagonists) or "antagonists at many receptors" (see Sect. 1.4) should be used. Implementation of these changes in terminology will take time. The term "antagonists at multiple G-protein-coupled receptors" does not make a classification that is nonexistent. Furthermore, it provides a better explanation as to why these drugs can be used for *many diseases* and why these drugs cause *many ADRs*.

Problems in Use of Antipsychotics

Because antipsychotics are antagonists at many different receptors, it is not surprising that they cause many ADRs (see Sect. 1.4). A reasonable compromise needs to be found between desired effects and ADRs in each patient. Therapeutic drug monitoring is important. Many patients with schizophrenia smoke tobacco. However, patients receiving antipsychotics should not smoke because tobacco constituents can accelerate breakdown of antipsychotics in the liver and thus reduce their effectiveness.

Most antipsychotics affect cardiovascular function. This is due to an antagonistic effect on alpha-1 receptors and/or muscarinic receptors. An antimuscarinic syndrome (including a dry mouth; GERD; hot, dry skin; a racing pulse; constipation; and urinary retention) may occur with all of these drugs except for haloperidol. Clozapine, olanzapine, quetiapine, and risperidone cause fatigue and increase appetite, leading to weight gain in long-term therapy. These two effects are due to antagonism at H_1 receptors (an antihistamine effect; see Sects. 4.1 and 9.2).

Clozapine

Clozapine is the most effective drug in schizophrenia, probably because of its antagonistic effects on so many receptors. Clozapine is the only antipsychotic that reduces suicidality in patients with schizophrenia and has a life-prolonging effect. Clozapine meets the most stringent criterion in clinical trials: prolongation of life (see Sect. 1.3). In addition, clozapine rarely causes movement disorders. All of the other drugs "only" improve quality of life.

There are three reasons why clozapine is not the undisputed gold standard in schizophrenia treatment, despite its compelling clinical efficacy:

1. Clozapine may cause dose-dependent depletion of white blood cells (agranulocytosis) in 1–2% of patients within the first 3 months of treatment, leading to increased susceptibility to infection.
2. Clozapine antagonizes more receptors than any other antipsychotic and therefore causes many ADRs (see Sect. 1.4). The most significant of these is marked weight gain (see Sect. 4.1) with a risk of development of type 2 diabetes (see Sect. 6.1) and correspondingly increased risks of high blood pressure, coronary heart disease, and strokes (see Sect. 5.1).

3. Clozapine is an inexpensive drug. From the pharmaceutical industry's point of view, not much money can be made from clozapine, which is why more lucrative drugs are advertised.

The clinical efficacy of clozapine was the reason for developing drugs that (1) are clinically just as effective but (2) do not cause agranulocytosis and (3) cause fewer ADRs overall. Unfortunately, only the second goal (no agranulocytosis) has been achieved. The newer antipsychotics olanzapine, quetiapine, and risperidone are not superior to clozapine, nor do they cause fewer ADRs (except for lack of agranulocytosis). They cause significantly more movement disorders than clozapine.

The risk of agranulocytosis with clozapine necessitates weekly blood counts at the start of treatment so that the dose can be reduced or the drug can be discontinued and replaced if necessary. Although agranulocytosis can be treated with white blood cell growth factors (see metamizole; Sect. 2.1), weekly clinic visits for a blood count require a high level of patient cooperation. For this reason, despite their lower efficacy, the three drugs olanzapine, quetiapine, and risperidone are preferred by many psychiatrists.

Other Uses of Antipsychotics

Antipsychotics are antagonists at many neurotransmitter receptors, causing numerous effects. It was therefore natural to try use of these drugs for other disorders besides schizophrenia. The first such use of antipsychotics was for acute mania (see Sect. 9.3). In addition, certain antipsychotics (especially haloperidol and risperidone) are effective in patients with cancer pain (see Sects. 2.2 and 11.1). Certain antipsychotics (especially haloperidol and olanzapine) have an antiemetic effect. This antiemetic effect is used to treat vomiting induced by cytostatics (see Sects. 3.1, 3.3, and 11.1). Antipsychotics are used for mental disorders such as depression (quetiapine and olanzapine; see Sect. 9.2), Tourette syndrome (quetiapine), autism (risperidone), obsessive–compulsive disorders (olanzapine, quetiapine, risperidone), and anxiety disorders (quetiapine). These areas of application show that the term "antipsychotics" is problematic.

Avoid Antipsychotics in Dementia

As a result of demographic changes, more people now suffer from dementia. Unfortunately, dementia can be treated only symptomatically. Antipsychotics such as haloperidol are used to "calm" agitated patients with dementia. However, this practice is ineffective and should be discontinued except in patients with hallucinations. It is dangerous for the following reasons:

1. Haloperidol does *not* have a sedative effect, as it lacks an antagonistic (antihistamine) effect on H_1 receptors.
2. Haloperidol can cause severe movement disorders, which can be misinterpreted as "sedation".
3. Haloperidol can cause severe hypotension, which can be misinterpreted as "sedation".
4. Haloperidol can cause severe arrhythmias, with a severely slowed heart rate. Misinterpretation as "sedation" is possible.
5. Because of points 2–4 (above), severe falls with dangerous bone fractures may occur, resulting in bed confinement with possible complications (e.g., pneumonia).

10

Drugs for Eye Diseases

Abstract Intact visual function is crucial for the independence of every person. This chapter deals with two important diseases leading to blindness: glaucoma and wet macular degeneration. Both represent diseases of old age. The first part of the chapter deals with glaucoma. Glaucoma is characterized by an imbalance between aqueous humor formation and outflow in the eye, causing intraocular pressure to rise. Various inexpensive drugs are available that, when used alone or in combination, can lower intraocular pressure and thus prevent progression of glaucoma. The second part of the chapter discusses wet macular degeneration. In this disease, fragile new blood vessels form in the choroid, burst, and cause bleeding. This can lead to rapid blindness. Progression of wet macular degeneration can be delayed with inhibitors of vessel formation that are injected into the vitreous body. The drugs approved for this purpose are expensive, but there are ways to save money.

10.1 Glaucoma

Summary

As a result of demographic changes, more people are suffering glaucoma, which can lead to blindness. Early detection and treatment of this disease are important. Glaucoma is caused by too much aqueous humor being produced and too little aqueous humor being discharged. As a result, intraocular pressure increases and damages the retina and the optic nerve. Prostaglandins are the most effective drugs for lowering intraocular pressure. They are used alone or in combination with alpha-2 receptor agonists, beta blockers, and carbonic anhydrase inhibitors. These drug classes can prevent blindness.

© The Author(s), under exclusive license to Springer Nature Switzerland AG 2022
R. Seifert, *Drugs Easily Explained*, https://doi.org/10.1007/978-3-031-12188-3_10

Memo

- Glaucoma can lead to blindness.
- Glaucoma can be effectively treated with drugs.
- Glaucoma therapy is monitored by intraocular pressure measurements.
- Prostaglandins are the most effective drug class used for treatment of glaucoma.
- Prostaglandins can cause eyelash elongation, iris discoloration, and skin discoloration around the eye.
- With use of different drug class combinations, almost every case of glaucoma can be treated.
- To avoid systemic adverse drug reactions (ADRs) after administration of eye drops, use your finger to press on the inner corner of the eye for 30–60 seconds.
- Antihistamines, antidepressants, and antipsychotics have parasympatholytic effects and can increase intraocular pressure.

What Is Glaucoma?

Glaucoma is a disorder mostly affecting old people. A key feature of glaucoma is an increase in intraocular pressure. In most cases of glaucoma, the increase in intraocular pressure goes unnoticed. As a result, the retina and the optic nerve become mechanically damaged. Initially, only the vision at the outer edges of the visual field is restricted. The visual field diminishes until the central vision is impaired. Finally, blindness occurs. Therefore, patients' independence and quality of life are massively restricted.

More than 50% of all patients with glaucoma do not receive appropriate drug treatment. The most important measures for early detection of glaucoma are regular visits to an ophthalmologist's or optometric's clinic for intraocular pressure measurement. Intraocular pressure is determined with a gauge placed on the cornea under short local anesthesia. Normal pressure values are between 10 and 21 millimeters of mercury (10–21 mmHg). Normal intraocular pressure does not exclude the presence of glaucoma. Unfortunately, once visual field loss has occurred, it cannot be reversed. In the best case, further visual field loss is delayed.

How Does Glaucoma Develop?

The aqueous humor is important for nutrition of the anterior parts of the eye (the lens, iris, and cornea) and can be thought of as a creek flowing from its source (aqueous humor formation) to its mouth (aqueous humor outflow).

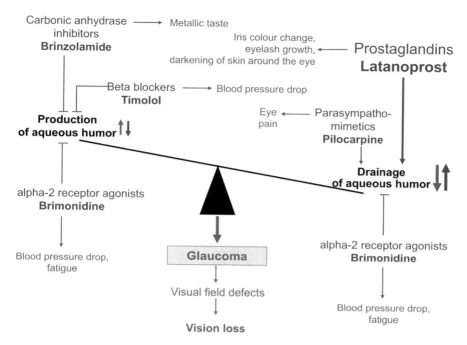

Fig. 10.1 How does glaucoma develop, and how is it treated? Glaucoma is character-ized by increased aqueous humor formation and reduced aqueous humor outflow. Since the eyeball is surrounded by a solid envelope (sclera), increased pressure cannot be buffered. Hence, intraocular pressure increases, and the subsequent retinal damage causes visual field loss and blindness. The aims of treatment are to inhibit formation of aqueous humor and/or increase outflow of aqueous humor. Prostaglandins (the proto-type drug is latanoprost) are the most effective drug class used for treatment of glau-coma. If this treatment is insufficient, different drug classes can be combined. This figure shows important adverse drug reactions (ADRs) associated with drugs used to treat glaucoma

Figure 10.1 shows the development of glaucoma and its treatment options. Table 10.1 gives an overview of the most important drug classes for treatment of glaucoma.

If too much aqueous humor is formed or if too little is drained, the humor backs up, intraocular pressure in the rigid eyeball increases, and glaucoma develops. This imbalance is the starting point for drug therapy: formation of aqueous humor is inhibited, while outflow of aqueous humor is increased.

Depending on whether the "mouth" of the aqueous humor flow is open or narrowed, a distinction is made between open-angle glaucoma and narrow-angle glaucoma. This is important for treatment.

Table 10.1 Overview of the most important drug classes used for treatment of glaucoma

Drug class	Prototype drug	Mechanisms of action	Indication	Important adverse drug reactions (ADRs) and interactions
Alpha-2 receptor agonists	**Brimonidine**	Reduce intraocular pressure by 25% by inhibiting aqueous humor formation and increasing aqueous humor outflow	Open-angle glaucoma (eye drops)	Blood pressure drop, fatigue
Beta blockers (beta receptor antagonists)	**Timolol**	Reduce intraocular pressure by 20–25% by inhibiting aqueous humor formation	Open-angle glaucoma (eye drops)	Blood pressure drop, heart rate decrease, asthma attacks
Carbonic anhydrase inhibitors	**Brinzolamide**	Reduces ocular pressure by approx. 20–25% by inhibiting aqueous humor formation	Open-angle glaucoma (eye drops); in cases of acute glaucoma, carbonic anhydrase inhibitors can be administered systemically	Metallic taste, risk of allergy
Parasympathomimetics (muscarine receptor agonists)	Pilocarpine	Facilitate outflow of aqueous humor by constricting the pupil	Narrow-angle glaucoma only	Eye pain, myopia; use restricted by ADRs
Prostaglandins (prostaglandin receptor agonists)	**Latanoprost**	Reduce intraocular pressure by up to 40% by strongly increasing outflow of aqueous humor	Open-angle glaucoma (eye drops); first-line drug class due to high efficacy	Irreversible iris discoloration; eyelash elongation; increased pigmentation (darkening) of skin around the eye; reduction of adipose tissue around the eye, resulting in a sunken eye appearance

Drug-specific word stems are shown in bold text. The drugs listed here are administered to the eye. This ensures a good local effect with comparatively minor ADRs. Systemic ADRs can be largely avoided by using a finger to press on the inner corner of the eye for approximately 30–60 seconds after application. This prevents the drug from entering the nose

ADR adverse drug reaction

The most common form of glaucoma is open-angle glaucoma. Its cause is unknown, but myopia, poorly controlled blood pressure (see Sect. 5.1), diabetes (see Sect. 6.1), and a family history of glaucoma are risk factors.

How Is Glaucoma Treated?

Increased intraocular pressure is the most important risk factor for development of glaucoma. Accordingly, the most important treatment goal in glaucoma is to reduce intraocular pressure. This significantly reduces the risk of long-term damage.

If glaucoma has damaged the eye, intraocular pressure must be reduced below "normal" values. Apart from emergencies such as acute glaucoma, the disease is treated with eye drops, so the effect of the drug can usually be limited to the eye. However, drugs administered to the eye can sometimes have systemic effects. This is because locally applied drugs can enter the nose through the eye–nasal canal. They can then be absorbed into the bloodstream through the mucous membranes of the nose. A simple precaution to prevent ADRs associated with glaucoma drugs applied outside the eye is to use your finger to press on the inner corner of the eye for 30–60 seconds after application of the drug.

Prostaglandins

Prostaglandins are the most effective drug class used for treatment of glaucoma. Their international nonproprietary names (INNs) can be recognized by the suffix "_prost" (the prototype drug is latanoprost). Prostaglandins reduce intraocular pressure by up to 40%. This effect is achieved by an increase in aqueous humor outflow. As a rule, prostaglandins are applied in the evening. Use of single-use eye drop containers reduces the risk of eye infections.

Unfortunately, prostaglandins can cause considerable ADRs. They can cause irreversible discoloration of the iris. In addition, prostaglandins can darken the skin around the eye, and the fatty tissue surrounding the eye can shrink. These changes are cosmetically disturbing.

Probably the best-known ADR associated with prostaglandins is that they lengthen the eyelashes. Many "natural serums" for eyelash elongation that are offered in beauty salons contain undeclared prostaglandins.

If prostaglandins are not effective for treatment of glaucoma or cannot be used because of ADRs, other drug classes are available. However, they are only about half as effective as prostaglandins, and different ADRs must be expected.

Alternatives to Prostaglandins

Like prostaglandins, alpha-2-receptor agonists increase outflow of aqueous humor. In addition, they reduce humor formation. The INNs of alpha-2 receptor agonists can be recognized by the suffix "_nidine". Brimonidine is a representative of this drug class. The main ADRs associated with alpha-2 receptor agonists are fatigue and low blood pressure. Therefore, in patients treated for high blood pressure, eye drops containing alpha-2 receptor agonists should be used only with caution. Otherwise, the blood pressure may drop too much.

Beta blockers lower intraocular pressure by reducing formation of aqueous humor. The INNs of this drug class can be recognized by the suffix "_olol". Timolol eye drops are frequently used to treat glaucoma. The properties of beta blockers are discussed in more detail in Sect. 5.1. The main ADRs associated with beta blockers are a drop in blood pressure, a reduced heart rate, and asthma attacks. Therefore, eye drops containing beta blockers should be used only with caution in patients receiving treatment for high blood pressure or asthma.

Carbonic anhydrase inhibitors are an alternative to the drug classes discussed above. They inhibit formation of aqueous humor. The INNs of carbonic anhydrase inhibitors can be recognized by the suffix "_zolamide". Brinzolamide is a representative of this drug class. Carbonic anhydrase inhibitors can cause a metallic taste. Sparkling wine and champagne no longer taste good ("champagne blues"). Therefore, to avoid this ADR, use your finger to press firmly on the inner corner of the eye for 30–60 seconds after applying a carbonic anhydrase inhibitor.

Various drug classes can be combined with each other to achieve a sufficient reduction in intraocular pressure. For most patients with glaucoma, it is possible to find suitable drug therapy with a good balance between therapeutic effects and ADRs. All of the drug classes discussed so far are used for open-angle glaucoma (which is common) and for narrow-angle glaucoma (which is rare). The parasympathomimetic pilocarpine is used only for narrow-angle glaucoma because it causes painful constriction of the pupil and myopia. Pilocarpine stimulates outflow of aqueous humor.

Which Drugs Can Worsen Glaucoma?

It is not only drugs that are administered to the eye that can cause systemic ADRs. Drugs that are supposed to act elsewhere in the body can affect the eye. The most important drugs with such effects are those that dilate the pupil and thus reduce aqueous humor outflow. As these drugs have the opposite effect to that of the parasympathomimetic (muscarinic receptor agonist) pilocarpine, they are called parasympatholytics (muscarinic receptor antagonists; see Sect. 1.4). Parasympatholytics dilate the pupil, increase intraocular pressure, and cause long-sightedness.

Parasympatholytics are used for a wide variety of conditions. They include biperiden, which is used in Parkinson's disease (see Sect. 8.1). Antidepressants from the group of nonselective monoamine reuptake inhibitors (NSMRIs; see Sect. 9.2), antipsychotics (see Sect. 9.4), and scopolamine (used for motion sickness [kinetosis]) can increase intraocular pressure through their parasympatholytic effect, as can high doses of antihistamines (see Sect. 4.1) and long-term glucocorticoid therapy (see Sect. 11.2).

What to Do in Acute Glaucoma

Acute glaucoma is an emergency. Massive visual disturbances in the affected eye, extreme eye pain, headaches, nausea, and vomiting are typical symptoms. Acute glaucoma usually develops on a background of inadequately treated glaucoma. Acute glaucoma can lead to blindness. If you are a glaucoma patient experiencing severe visual disturbances and a headache, go to an eye clinic immediately!

Acute glaucoma must be treated immediately with the drug classes discussed above. In addition, carbonic anhydrase inhibitors can be given intravenously. Finally, intraocular pressure can be lowered by use of strong dehydrating drugs such as mannitol. However, these drugs cause severe ADRs. If drug therapy is ineffective, surgical procedures are used. The best treatment for acute glaucoma is its prevention.

10.2   Wet Macular Degeneration

Summary

Wet macular degeneration is a common cause of blindness in old people. In this disease, a growth factor is released in the choroid of the eye, leading to uncontrolled growth of fragile new blood vessels. These vessels can burst and cause bleeding, leading to blindness. Wet macular degeneration can be treated with drugs, (injected into the vitreous body of the eye), that inhibit growth factors. Aflibercept and ranibizumab are two drugs approved for treatment of wet macular degeneration, but they are expensive. Bevacizumab is equally effective but is not approved for treatment of wet macular degeneration. Nevertheless, off-label treatment with bevacizumab is an alternative.

Memo

- An acute change in visual acuity or "distorted vision" may be an indication of macular degeneration.
- In wet macular degeneration, new blood vessels develop and can burst.
- Prevention of new blood vessel formation is the most important principle in treatment of wet macular degeneration.
- The blood vessel growth inhibitors aflibercept, ranibizumab, and bevacizumab are similarly effective, but bevacizumab is much less expensive.

What Is Macular Degeneration?

Macular degeneration is a disease of old age. The macula (yellow spot) is the place of sharpest vision on the retina. When a disease occurs there, all everyday activities are severely affected. Two forms of macular degeneration are distinguished. In dry macular degeneration, pigments are deposited in the macula. Although 80% of all cases of macular degeneration are classified as the dry form, it rarely causes blindness. Wet macular degeneration is much more dangerous. This disease accounts for only 20% of all cases of macular degeneration but almost all cases of blindness. An early symptom of wet macular degeneration is distorted perception of grid lines and writing. Other early symptoms of wet macular degeneration are sensitivity to glare and reduced ability to perceive contrasts. An ophthalmologist can diagnose dry or wet macular degeneration with ophthalmoscopy.

How Does Wet Macular Degeneration Develop?

Figure 10.2 shows the development of wet macular degeneration and its treatment. Poorly controlled high blood pressure (see Sect. 5.1), exposure to ultraviolet (UV) light, tobacco consumption, and advanced age contribute to development of wet macular degeneration.

In wet macular degeneration, vascular endothelial growth factor (VEGF) is released in large quantities in the choroid. The choroid has many blood

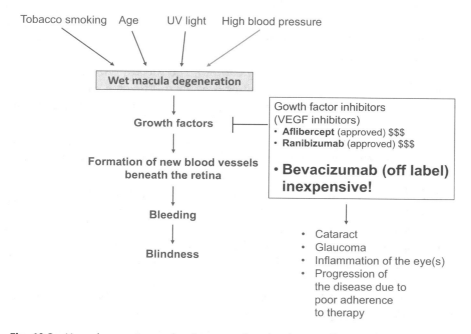

Fig. 10.2 How does wet macular degeneration develop, and how is it treated? There are a number of preventable causes (high blood pressure [see Sect. 5.1], exposure to ultraviolet light, and tobacco smoking) of development of wet macular degeneration, which is characterized by increased production of growth factors in the choroid. These growth factors trigger formation of fragile new blood vessels. When these blood vessels burst, bleeding occurs, which can lead to acute blindness. Thus, the most effective treatment for this disease is to inhibit the action of growth factors with inhibitors (vascular endothelial growth factor [VEGF] inhibitors). Aflibercept, ranibizumab, and bevacizumab have similar efficacy and are associated with similar adverse drug reactions (ADRs). Only aflibercept and ranibizumab are approved for treatment of wet macular degeneration. It is up to you as a patient to contribute to cost control in health care systems by agreeing to treatment with the equally effective but much less expensive drug bevacizumab. This figure shows important ADRs associated with the three VEGF inhibitors

vessels, which are responsible for nourishing the retina, where the process of vision takes place.

VEGF is normally useful in the body. It ensures that small blood vessels (capillaries) are formed. Capillaries supply our body cells with oxygen and nutrients. With too much VEGF in the choroid, many vessels sprout. Unfortunately, these new vessels lack a well-developed vessel wall. Therefore, they can burst, and bleeding can occur. The bleeding can flood the choroid and the retina. Rapid blindness can be the result.

How Is Wet Macular Degeneration Treated?

Acute bleeding in the choroid must be treated immediately. This is mainly done with high-energy lasers. The laser beams locally destroy the affected parts of the retina and the underlying choroid, and thereby close the ruptured vessels. However, laser therapy does not prevent misdirected new vessel formation. After laser therapy for wet macular degeneration, fragile vessels can form again and new bleeding can occur.

The goal of therapy is to neutralize VEGF and thus prevent formation of fragile new vessels. Long-term treatment is required. VEGF inhibitors are not suitable to stop acute bleeding. VEGF inhibitors are either soluble receptors for VEGF or antibodies that bind VEGF and thus prevent vessel growth. Since VEGF inhibitors are proteins, they must be injected into the vitreous body. The injection is given under local anesthesia with an ultrafine needle through the sclera of the eye (the white part of the eye). From the vitreous body, the VEGF inhibitors diffuse into the choroid and inhibit growth of fragile vessels.

Two drugs are approved for treatment of wet macular degeneration: the soluble VEGF receptor aflibercept and the "mini" antibody ranibizumab. In these INNs, the suffix "_cept" stands for "soluble receptor" and the suffix "_mab" stands for "monoclonal antibody". The effects of VEGF inhibitors slowly wear off; thus, these drugs must be regularly reinjected into the vitreous body every 4–12 weeks. If an appointment for a VEGF inhibitor injection is not kept, the risk of bleeding increases.

Adverse Drug Reactions Associated with Vascular Endothelial Growth Factor Inhibitors

Injection of a drug into the vitreous body must be done under sterile conditions. Otherwise, infections can occur inside the eye. Since the eye is not readily accessible to antibiotics, penetration of the eye by bacteria can lead to blindness. In addition, injection of VEGF inhibitors can lead to cataracts and glaucoma (see Sect. 10.1). Therefore, both regular examinations of the anterior segment of the eye with a slit lamp (to detect lens opacities [cataracts]) and intraocular pressure measurements (to detect glaucoma) are required.

Bevacizumab as an Alternative to Aflibercept and Bevacizumab

Treatment with an approved VEGF inhibitor costs several thousand dollars per year. The high therapy costs of aflibercept and ranibizumab represent a significant financial problem for health care systems globally. However, another VEGF inhibitor (bevacizumab) is approved for treatment of various cancers (see Sect. 11.1). The "maxi" antibody bevacizumab is much less expensive than ranibizumab. Both antibodies are marketed by the same company. It argues that ranibizumab was specifically developed for use in the eye and that because of its smaller ("mini") size, this drug reaches the choroid more easily than the "maxi" drug bevacizumab.

Many clinical trials have been conducted to compare the efficacy of aflibercept, ranibizumab, and bevacizumab. All three drugs have comparable efficacy in wet macular degeneration and are associated with similar ADRs. Thus, aflibercept, ranibizumab, and bevacizumab are interchangeable for treatment of wet macular degeneration. If all patients with wet macular degeneration were treated with bevacizumab instead of the other two drugs, the therapy costs would be only a fraction of the current costs.

This situation poses a dilemma for eye doctors: Do they act for the sake of society and treat their patients with an effective and inexpensive drug without approval for its use in wet macular degeneration, or do they use an effective and expensive drug that is approved for use in this disease?

Often the problem is solved by applying bevacizumab "off-label" (i.e., without approval for treatment of wet macular degeneration). Off-label treatments of other drugs are commonly used in mental disorders (see Sects. 1.3, 9.1, and 9.4). However, the liability risk in the event of an ADR lies with the doctor. For this reason, many ophthalmologists are reluctant to prescribe bevacizumab off-label.

It is to be hoped that when the patent protection for bevacizumab expires, new suppliers will come onto the market with inexpensive bevacizumab generics for treatment of wet macular degeneration. The examples of ranibizumab and bevacizumab show how pharmaceutical manufacturers can exploit their market position to maximize profits. If you are a patient with wet macular degeneration, you can contribute to cost reduction in health care systems by agreeing to have it treated off-label with bevacizumab.

11

Drugs for Cancer and for Autoimmune and Infectious Diseases

Abstract This chapter provides an overview of treatment options for cancers, autoimmune diseases, and infectious diseases. In cancer, in addition to classic chemotherapy, new drugs are used to target malignant cells more specifically. Good pain management is crucial in cancer therapy. Glucocorticoids (known colloquially as "cortisone") are still the most important class of drugs used for autoimmune diseases. A major problem in treatment of infectious diseases is use of antibiotics without proper indication. This results in development of resistance and consequent lack of treatment options for severe infections.

11.1 Cancer

Summary

Cancers (malignant diseases) are a common cause of death globally. Cancers are the result of gene mutations, environmental factors, and viruses. Cancer cells multiply uncontrollably and destroy organs. Treatment with cytostatics takes advantage of the fact that cancer cells grow rapidly. However, cytostatics additionally damage fast-growing normal body cells. A new approach to cancer treatment is use of targeted therapeutics to inhibit cancer growth more specifically. The adverse drug reactions (ADRs) associated with targeted therapeutics differ from those caused by cytostatics. To prevent cancer cells from developing resistance, cytostatics are combined with targeted therapeutics.

Memo

- Cancers (malignant diseases) are the result of gene mutations.
- Cancer cells grow rapidly.
- Rapid growth of cancer cells is exploited in chemotherapy with cytostatics.
- Cytostatics lead to hair loss, blood formation disorders, and mucosal damage.
- Vomiting induced by cytostatics is controlled with serotonin-3 receptor antagonists.
- Targeted therapeutics inhibit cancer cell growth more specifically than cytostatics.
- The ADRs associated with targeted therapeutics differ from those caused by cytostatics.
- Cytostatics are combined with targeted therapeutics.
- Good pain management is crucial in cancer therapy (see Chap. 2), particularly in patients with terminal cancer.

What Is Cancer?

"Cancer" is a colloquial term for malignant diseases. Cancer cells grow uncontrollably, eat their way into normal tissue, and cause daughter tumors (metastases). The faster a cancer grows, the better it can usually be treated. If the cancer is not detected in time, the patient is more likely to die, especially from metastases.

Depending on the malignant cells from which the cancer originates, we distinguish between carcinomas (which originate in epithelial cells), sarcomas (which originate in connective tissue), and malignancies of the hematopoietic system (leukemia or lymphoma). In women, mammary carcinoma (breast cancer) is the most common cancer, followed by bronchial carcinoma (lung cancer) and colon carcinoma. In men, the most common cancer is bronchial carcinoma, followed by colon carcinoma and prostate carcinoma (prostate cancer).

Cancer Development

Figure 11.1 shows an overview of the development of cancer and principles of drug therapy. The common feature of all malignant diseases is uncontrolled cell growth.

Growth of normal body cells is tightly controlled. Gene mutations disrupt these control mechanisms in cancer. Some gene mutations are inherited (i.e., certain cancers have a familial predisposition). A variety of external factors can lead to gene mutations. These include chemicals (e.g., asbestos, benzene, and

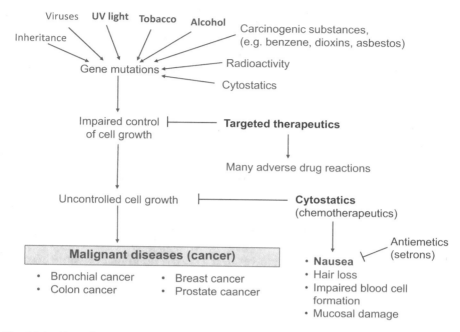

Fig. 11.1   How do cancers develop, and how are they treated? Many factors can cause development of cancer. You can make important contributions to prevention of cancer development: skin cancer can be prevented by minimizing exposure to strong ultraviolet (UV) radiation (with use of sun protection), and development of oral and tongue cancer is prevented by avoiding tobacco and alcohol. Tobacco is the most important cause of lung cancer. Cytostatics (chemotherapeutics) inhibit uncontrolled cell growth but additionally inhibit growth of rapidly growing normal body cells, resulting in severe adverse drug reactions (ADRs). Nausea is particularly distressing but can be treated with serotonin-3 receptor antagonists (setrons). Many targeted therapeutics for specific cancer types are on the market. Cytostatics are combined with targeted therapeutics

dioxin), exposure to strong ultraviolet (UV) radiation, heavy alcohol consumption, tobacco use, and exposure to radioactive radiation. Viruses (e.g., hepatitis C virus) can cause cancer. The most common cause of cancer is tobacco consumption, which mainly causes lung and mouth cancers. Cytostatics themselves can trigger cancer many years after being successfully used in initial treatment. This is referred to as secondary cancer.

Cancer Diagnostics and Treatment

Diagnosis of malignant diseases has traditionally been focused on the fine structure (histology). In addition, attention is paid to the size of the primary tumor (T), the number of lymph nodes (N) that are affected, and the number of metastases (M). This approach is known as the TNM (Tumor–Node–Metastasis) system. Histological tumor diagnosis and the TNM system are still valid, but another dimension has now been added for treatment: in many tumor types, gene mutations that control cell growth are now analyzed.

When the cancer diagnosis has been established, a "tumor conference" is held. At this conference, doctors from various specialties come together and decide what the best treatment approach is for each patient they are caring for. In most cases, surgical and pharmacological treatments are combined. For some cancers, radiation with high-energy ionizing radiation and/or administration of radioactive substances (see Sect. 6.2) are used. Nowadays, cancer treatment has become so specialized that it would go far beyond the scope of this book to discuss individual types of cancer; instead, the principles of cancer therapy are discussed here. The goal is to cure the patient of their cancer. This is called curative therapy. However, if a cure is no longer possible because the cancer has progressed too far, palliative treatment is used. The aims of palliative treatment are to prolong survival and improve the quality of life.

Cytostatics

Cytostatics attack the cell cycle (cell division) and stop tumor cell growth. Many cytostatics damage the DNA (deoxyribonucleic acid) of the cancer cells. In most cases, several cytostatics with different mechanisms of action are combined to increase the effectiveness of the cancer therapy and to prevent cancer cells from becoming resistant to it. Resistance develops because malignant cells have effective mechanisms for "throwing out" (exporting) cytostatics. The more different cytostatics a cancer is treated with, the more difficult it is for the malignant cells to throw out the cytostatics and thus become resistant. This treatment strategy improves the prognosis of the cancer patient in terms of their quality of life and survival time.

Many cytostatics irritate blood vessels. Therefore, cancer patients are given a "port" (central venous catheter). This port allows the drugs to be infused into a large blood vessel without causing blood vessel irritation.

Cytostatics are administered in cycles interrupted by breaks. This approach serves to improve the tolerability of the treatment and to promote the recovery of the body. Modern cancer treatment has lost much of its previous horror, and more patients are being cured. A "cure" is defined as the patient having no detectable relapse for at least 5 years after their initial cancer diagnosis. However, the term "cured" is not synonymous with "healthy", because the cytostatics used to treat the cancer may have caused gene mutations in the patient's healthy body cells, which later can lead to secondary cancers.

Adverse Drug Reactions due to Cytostatics

Cytostatic drugs cause a fatigue syndrome. A good way of treating fatigue syndrome is to do mild exercise within the limits of what is possible. Walks have a positive effect on well-being.

Cytostatics cause nausea and vomiting. This ADR is unpleasant and can lead to severe water and salt losses. In the past, vomiting was an ADR that limited cytostatic treatment. Nowadays, several drug classes can be used (alone or in combination) to treat cytostatic-induced vomiting. The most effective class of drugs for this purpose are serotonin-3 receptor antagonists (setrons), which allow many patients to receive cancer treatment on an outpatient basis. Many antipsychotic drugs have antiemetic effects as well (see Sect. 9.4).

Cytostatics do not distinguish between cancer cells and healthy body cells. They inhibit growth of fast-growing normal cells, resulting in loss of hair. Mucous membranes, which are rapidly renewed, are impaired in their function as well. The most prominent symptoms are burning of the mouth and tongue, esophageal burns, and diarrhea. Bone marrow is damaged, which results in a drop in the white blood cell count and thus increases susceptibility to infections with bacteria, viruses, and fungi (see Sect. 11.3). The numbers of red blood cells, which are responsible for transporting oxygen to the organs, decrease too. Patients therefore often look pale and have limited physical capacity. Finally, the blood platelet count can also drop, which can lead to more severe bleeding after injuries. If children must be treated with cytostatics, this can lead to growth retardation and ultimately a reduced body size.

Cytostatics and Childbearing

An important problem for cancer patients who wish to have children is that cytostatics have mutagenic effects on germ cells. Unfortunately, this ADR cannot be avoided, because it is this mechanism that destroys cancer cells. If time permits, cancer patients who wish to have children can have their oocytes or sperm cells harvested prior to cytostatic therapy and frozen for later in vitro fertilization.

Cytostatics have damaging effects on the embryo and fetus. However, if a pregnant woman needs cancer treatment, this is not a reason to terminate the pregnancy. Modern therapy makes it possible for women with cancer to give birth to healthy children.

Targeted Therapeutics

The development of targeted therapeutics was driven by two different factors. First, the ADRs caused by cytostatics put pressure on doctors, researchers, and the pharmaceutical industry to develop better-tolerated drugs. Second, research into the biology of cancer cells opened up new possibilities for drug development. Targeted therapeutics specifically turn off mechanisms that control cancer cell growth. Depending on the targeted therapeutic that is used, ADRs range from accumulation of white blood cells in the lungs to skin rashes, high blood pressure, wound healing disorders, and hot flashes. However, it would go too far to discuss the individual ADRs associated with each targeted therapeutic here.

Development of targeted therapeutics for cancer is currently one of the most active areas of drug development. As a result, treatment of individual types of cancer can be improved. Unfortunately, targeted therapeutics have become one of the biggest cost drivers in health care systems. In various cases, it is doubtful whether the high drug prices are justified.

In the examples described below, three principles of targeted therapeutics are described.

Example 1: Starving Cancer Cells

One of the most important factors for rapid cancer growth is adequate supply of oxygen and nutrients to the cancer. For this purpose, a cancer needs blood vessels. Many tumors stimulate formation of blood vessels by releasing growth factors. With the help of antibodies (e.g., bevacizumab; see Sect. 10.2), it is possible to disable these growth factors and thus stop growth of blood vessels in the cancer. The cancer is thereby "starved". This treatment approach is applied in many advanced cancers. A disadvantage is that formation of new normal blood vessels is inhibited as well. This can lead to an increase in blood pressure (see Sect. 5.1) or vascular occlusion (see Sect. 5.2).

Example 2: Inhibiting Growth Factors in Breast Cancer

Some cancer cells have receptors for growth factors that stimulate growth of cancer cells. For example, the human epidermal growth factor (EGF) increases growth of breast cancer cells through a specific receptor known as HER2 (human epidermal growth factor receptor 2). The function of this receptor is inhibited by a specific antibody (trastuzumab). To find out whether a patient with breast cancer can benefit from trastuzumab, it must be checked whether the cancer cells carry this receptor. Trastuzumab can cause allergies, susceptibility to infections, headaches, insomnia, and heart failure.

> **Example 3: Blocking Estrogen Receptors in Breast Cancer**
>
> When breast cancer cells have estrogen receptors (see Sect. 7.1), estrogen can promote growth of those cells. Tamoxifen, a selective estrogen receptor modulator (SERM), blocks the growth-promoting effect of estrogen on breast cancer cells but stimulates estrogen receptors in the uterus, the heart/circulatory system, and the bones. Tamoxifen can cause unpleasant ADRs such as hot flashes and weight gain. Before treatment with tamoxifen, it must be checked whether the breast cancer cells carry estrogen receptors.

Pain Management

Often it is not possible to cure a cancer patient. Pain is caused by local growth of cancer and metastases. Bone metastases are particularly painful. At this stage of incurable cancer, palliative pain treatment plays a major role. It allows patients to have a good quality of life and to remain at home. The goal for the patient is to be pain-free. Palliative medicine has made progress in recent years. It is possible to find good pain therapy at the last stage of life for most patients.

In accordance with the World Health Organization (WHO) pain management plan, nonopioid analgesics (see Sect. 2.1) are initially used, with consideration of the patient's individual situation and ADRs. At the second stage, weak opioid analgesics (first tramadol, then buprenorphine) are added. At the third stage, strong opioid analgesics such as morphine and fentanyl (see Sect. 2.2) are administered. Patients may self-administer opioid analgesics (e.g., fentanyl nasal spray or fentanyl lozenges) for pain peaks, within certain limits. Palliative pain therapy does not cause opioid addiction. At the final stage, pump systems delivering analgesics under the skin (subcutaneously) or intravenously are frequently used.

Additional drug classes are used as "coanalgesics" at all stages of the WHO pain management plan. For pain caused by bone metastases, bisphosphonates and denosumab are particularly effective (see Sect. 6.3). Nonselective monoamine reuptake inhibitors (NSMRIs; the prototype drug is amitriptyline), which belong to the antidepressant drug class, are particularly effective for nerve pain (see Sect. 9.2). Antipsychotics (the prototype drug is haloperidol; see Sect. 9.3) distance the patient from the pain. Many antipsychotics work well against nausea and vomiting at the same time, complementing the effects of setrons. Benzodiazepines support pain management through their sleep-inducing, sedative, and anxiolytic effects (see Sect. 8.2). In addition, various antiepileptic drugs (see Sect. 8.2) and the glutamate inhibitor ketamine (see

Sects. 2.1 and 8.2) are used in treatment of cancer pain. Ketamine has antidepressant effects (see Sect. 8.1) as well as sedative, sleep-inducing, and analgesic effects.

Ingredients of hemp (*Cannabis sativa*) are promoted for palliative cancer therapy. Dronabinol is the prototypical representative of the cannabis ingredients. It activates cannabinoid receptors in the brain as an agonist (see Sect. 1.4). Dronabinol inhibits nausea and vomiting, increases appetite, and has sleep-inducing, mild analgesic, and muscle-relaxing effects. However, the outcome of clinical trials on the efficacy of cannabis ingredients in cancer patients has been disappointing; thus, prescribing of cannabis preparations is not recommended.

11.2   Autoimmune Diseases

Summary

Normally, the body does not attack its own cells. However, in autoimmune diseases, the body directs an immune reaction against its own cells. This leads to symptoms of inflammation (pain, swelling, and redness) and, ultimately, loss of function of the affected organ. The cause of autoimmune diseases is unknown. Treatment of these diseases is symptomatic and focuses on inhibition of certain white blood cells (T cells) and release of mediators of inflammation. The most important and versatile drugs are the glucocorticoids (known colloquially as "cortisone"). In addition, numerous special drugs are used. By use of combinations of drugs, many autoimmune diseases can be controlled.

Memo

- In autoimmune diseases, an immune reaction against the patient's own body is mounted.
- Drug therapy for autoimmune diseases is symptomatic.
- Often, an autoimmune disease requires lifelong treatment.
- Glucocorticoids (cortisone) are the most important drugs for autoimmune diseases.
- When glucocorticoids are used properly, the ADRs associated with them are acceptable.
- Many drugs used for autoimmune diseases increase susceptibility to infection.
- Low-dose methotrexate (MTX) is suitable for autoimmune diseases.
- MTX is given only once a week!
- Chloroquine works well in lupus erythematosus.

What Are Autoimmune Diseases?

The most important task of our immune system is to distinguish between the body's own cells and "foreign" cells (invading bacteria, viruses, and fungi; see Sect. 11.3). When the immune system receives the signal "foreign", it mounts an inflammatory response with the aim of destroying the invading pathogens and restoring health. If the immune system does not function properly (e.g., in the case of certain hereditary diseases or because of administration of cytostatics; see Sect. 11.1), susceptibility to infections increases.

Normally, the distinction between the body's own cells and foreign cells works. In autoimmune diseases, however, this distinction breaks down, with a subsequent attack of the immune system on the body. This self-destructive attack results in symptoms of inflammation (pain, swelling, and redness) and, ultimately, loss of function (or, in rare instances, hyperfunction; see Sect. 6.2) of the specific organ. In some autoimmune diseases (type 1 diabetes [see Sect. 6.1] and hyperthyroidism or hypothyroidism [see Sect. 6.2]), the organ dysfunction can be treated directly. Figure 11.2 shows the development of autoimmune diseases and targets for drug therapy.

The cause of autoimmune diseases is unknown. Therefore, they can be treated only symptomatically. The immune system is suppressed to alleviate the symptoms of the disease. Autoimmune diseases often require lifelong treatment, and susceptibility to infections is increased.

Any Organ Can Be Affected

Any organ can be affected by an autoimmune disease. Rheumatoid arthritis primarily affects joints and ulcerative colitis affects the rectum, while Crohn disease affects the entire gastrointestinal tract. Psoriasis mainly affects the skin. A common feature of these diseases is that they are systemic. Although these diseases have a main organ where their symptoms appear, the disease can spread to other organs. For example, inflammation of the joints is often found in psoriasis, and inflammation of the eyes (iritis) occurs in rheumatoid arthritis and Crohn disease. Lupus erythematosus is a systemic autoimmune disease that primarily affects the skin or kidneys. When it affects the kidneys, it often leads to high blood pressure (see Sect. 5.1) and ultimately to kidney failure. The most important autoimmune disease of the brain is multiple sclerosis, which is usually a relapsing condition and begins at a young age.

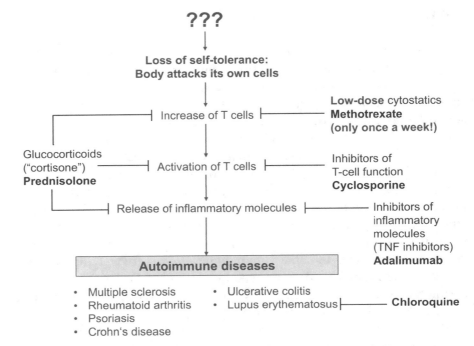

Fig. 11.2 How do autoimmune diseases develop, and how are they treated? The cause of autoimmune diseases is unknown. After breakdown of tolerance against the body's own cells, a multistage process involving T cells leads to inflammation. Any organ can be affected. Autoimmune diseases can be treated only symptomatically. Attempts are made to inhibit various stages of the inflammatory process. Glucocorticoids such as prednisolone (known colloquially as "cortisone") are still the most important drugs. Many other drugs are available for treatment of autoimmune diseases. Of particular importance are certain cytostatics (see Sect. 11.1), given in low doses

T Cells as a Focus of Therapy

Because of breakdown of self-tolerance, the number of T cells (a certain type of white blood cells) increases. (The "T" in the term "T cell" refers to the thymus (a type of large lymph node behind the breastbone), from which these cells originate.) Once the T cells multiply, they are activated and release many mediators of inflammation that initiate a self-destructive autoimmune process and lead to clinical symptoms. Depending on the type of autoimmune disease, different mediators of inflammation are involved. Accordingly, each autoimmune disease is treated somewhat differently. Most drugs used for treatment of autoimmune diseases attack T cells directly or indirectly (see Fig. 11.2).

"Cortisone" and Nonsteroidal Anti-inflammatory Drugs

Rheumatoid arthritis is the classic autoimmune disease. Many of the treatment concepts for autoimmune diseases were developed on the basis of this paradigm. Until the 1950s, there were hardly any options for treating rheumatoid arthritis. Then clinical trials found that the hormone hydrocortisone (cortisol) had good anti-inflammatory (antiphlogistic) effects in rheumatoid arthritis. The term "hydrocortisone" then became colloquially abbreviated as "cortisone".

However, it soon emerged that hydrocortisone not only had therapeutic effects but also could cause serious ADRs such as peptic ulcer disease (PUD; see Sect. 3.1), high blood pressure and weight gain (see Sect. 5.1), diabetes (see Sect. 6.1), and osteoporosis (see Sect. 6.3). Cortisone was therefore discredited as being dangerous, and this bad reputation has persisted to the present day.

Cortisone belongs to the steroid hormones, as do sex hormones (see Sect. 7.1). Because of the ADRs that "steroids" can cause, attempts were made to develop "nonsteroidal" anti-inflammatory drugs in the hope that they would be better tolerated than "steroidal" anti-inflammatory drugs (cortisone). The results of this development were the nonsteroidal anti-inflammatory drugs (NSAIDs), with the prototype drugs being diclofenac and ibuprofen (see Sect. 2.1). Indeed, these drugs showed good anti-inflammatory effects in rheumatoid arthritis, and at first it looked as if NSAIDs would be a good alternative to cortisone, as the term "nonsteroidal" suggested. However, it became apparent that with long-term use, NSAIDs can cause severe ADRs that overlap with those caused by cortisone. These include a risk of PUD (see Sect. 3.2), risks of high blood pressure and kidney failure (see Sects. 2.1 and 5.1), and asthma (see Sect. 4.1). NSAIDs nonselectively inhibit cyclooxygenases (COXs) and thus inhibit formation of prostaglandin E (PGE). This mechanism produces the desired analgesic and anti-inflammatory effects but also causes the ADRs (see Sect. 2.1).

Disease-Modifying Antirheumatic Drugs

These sobering results were the starting point for a search for anti-inflammatory drugs that caused neither the ADRs associated with cortisone nor those associated with NSAIDs. These newer anti-inflammatory drugs were called "disease-modifying antirheumatic drugs" (DMARDs). However, this is an umbrella term for diverse drugs; it has never been clearly defined which drugs are DMARDs. Moreover, many DMARDs were found to cause serious ADRs. Many of the formerly used DMARDs have since become irrelevant because of insufficient efficacy and severe ADRs.

An exception is chloroquine. It was developed for prophylaxis and treatment of malaria. Because of the increasing resistance of malaria pathogens and development of more effective and better-tolerated drugs, the importance of chloroquine as an antimalarial drug has greatly diminished. In the search for DMARDs, it was discovered by chance that chloroquine is effective in rheumatoid arthritis and especially in lupus erythematosus. The mechanism of action of chloroquine is not known. The most common ADRs are arrhythmias, visual disturbances, nerve damage, nausea, and vomiting.

Coxibs

Later, attempts were made to selectively inhibit cyclooxygenase-2 (COX-2) because COX-2 was thought to be involved only in inflammatory processes. But this is not true, because COX-2 also plays a major role in cardiovascular function. Long-term use of COX-2 inhibitors (the prototype drug is etoricoxib) is associated with increased risks of strokes and heart attacks (see Sects. 2.1 and 5.2). For these reasons, NSAIDs and coxibs should be used only for a short time. In some countries, coxibs are not approved at all because of the ADRs they can cause.

Treatment of Autoimmune Diseases with Cortisone

The disadvantage of cortisone is that this hormone is equally effective at glucocorticoid receptors and at mineralocorticoid receptors. Glucocorticoid receptors mediate the anti-inflammatory effects, the metabolic effects (diabetes [see Sect. 6.1], osteoporosis [see Sect. 6.3], and muscle wasting), and the effects on the stomach (PUD; see Sect. 3.2), while mineralocorticoid receptors mediate the cardiovascular effects (high blood pressure and weight gain; see Sect. 5.1). Nowadays, cortisone derivatives such as prednisolone are used to treat autoimmune diseases. Prednisolone has significantly fewer effects on the cardiovascular system at a dose that exhibits similar anti-inflammatory effects.

The good effect of prednisolone on autoimmune diseases is due to inhibition of T cells and release of mediators of inflammation. The effects of prednisolone start 12–18 hours after its intake. This is because prednisolone affects cellular processes at the gene level, which takes time (see Sect. 1.4). The effect of prednisolone lasts for 18–36 hours. The advantages of the slow onset and the long-lasting effect of prednisolone are that there are no fluctuations in efficacy, which is important for adherence to treatment.

Prednisolone causes fewer ADRs in the cardiovascular system than cortisone. To minimize ADRs, high-dose treatment with prednisolone is no longer given over a long period. Instead, the treatment starts with a high dose, which is reduced as quickly as possible. The prednisolone dose is adapted on the basis of the patient's clinical symptoms and laboratory parameters. The aim is to find an optimal balance between the anti-inflammatory effect and ADRs.

Another important rule is to take prednisolone in the morning. This fits the daily rhythm of cortisone release and makes it easier for endogenous cortisone production to resume when prednisolone is stopped. It is important to taper off the prednisolone dosage over a period of weeks. If the patient adheres to these rules, systemic treatment with prednisolone in low doses can be carried out for a long time if needed.

Treatment with prednisolone requires regular checkups; blood pressure, kidney function, blood glucose concentrations, and bone density must be controlled. Use of a proton pump inhibitor may be needed to prevent PUD (see Sect. 3.2). Osteoporosis can be avoided by consumption of a diet rich in vitamin D and calcium (see Sect. 6.3). Type 2 diabetes does not occur with a healthy diet and adequate exercise. Endurance exercise and strength training counteract muscle wasting. Prednisolone increases susceptibility to infections (see Sect. 11.3). In ulcerative colitis, the risk of ADRs is reduced by application of the drug budesonide as a rectal foam. Budesonide acts only locally because it is immediately broken down in the liver after absorption into the bloodstream (see Sect. 1.5).

Low-Dose Cytostatics

Although modern treatment of autoimmune diseases with prednisolone is effective, the ADRs it causes necessitate use of additional drug classes to control autoimmune diseases. From cancer therapy, it was learned that cytostatics weaken the immune system and increase susceptibility to infection (see Sect. 11.1). This effect was exploited in autoimmune diseases by reducing the doses of cytostatics. A single, very low dose of the cytostatic methotrexate per week—just a hundredth (1%) of the corresponding weekly dose used for cancer—improves many autoimmune diseases. The ADRs associated with cytostatic treatment (such as hair loss, nausea, and vomiting; see Sect. 11.1) do not occur with low-dose MTX treatment.

Risks Associated with Low-Dose Methotrexate

1. MTX is given only once a week, *not* daily. Cooperation of the patient is essential. Otherwise, an accidental MTX overdose could easily occur in the event of a change of doctor or hospitalization.
2. Blood counts must be performed regularly, as MTX can impair blood cell formation.
3. It is important to check for signs of infection (see Sect. 11.3).
4. Kidney function must be controlled. With impaired kidney function, excretion of MTX is reduced (see Sect. 1.5). Accordingly, the MTX dosage must be reduced.
5. Coadministration of other renally excreted drugs such as NSAIDs (see Sect. 2.1) delays excretion of MTX and thus increases its toxicity.

Many deaths from low-dose MTX have occurred because these precautions were not taken. As an alternative to MTX, cyclophosphamide or azathioprine (6-mercaptopurine) can be given in a low dose to control autoimmune diseases.

Treatment of Autoimmune Diseases with Inhibitors of T Cell Function

Ciclosporin was the first drug used to specifically inhibit the function of T cells. Ciclosporin blocks formation of interleukin-2 (IL-2), which is of importance for activation of T cells. The drug is effective in many autoimmune diseases and prevention of transplant rejection. Ciclosporin was the starting point for development of several other drugs that inhibit T cell function. These include everolimus and tacrolimus. These three drugs differ from each other in terms of the ADRs associated with them; thus, patients can be offered alternatives among them.

Specific (and Expensive) Approaches

Research in the 1980s and 1990s showed that, in addition to the well-known "players" PGE and IL-2, other mediators of inflammation play important roles in many autoimmune diseases. These include tumor necrosis factor (TNF) and the interleukins IL-6, IL-12, and IL-23. Many antibodies are now available that can block these mediators of inflammation and thus reduce inflammatory symptoms in autoimmune diseases. The antibodies are injected under the skin (subcutaneously) at intervals of several weeks to months. However, treatment with these antibodies is much more expensive than prednisolone treatment.

TNF inhibitors show good efficacy in rheumatoid arthritis, Crohn's disease, and ulcerative colitis, and they are alternatives to glucocorticoids and low-dose cytostatics. However, TNF inhibitors increase susceptibility to infection (see Sect. 11.3) and worsen heart failure (see Sect. 5.3). IL-6 inhibitors (e.g., tocilizumab) are used in rheumatoid arthritis. IL-12/IL-23 inhibitors (e.g., ustekinumab) are used in psoriasis and Crohn's disease.

11.3 Infectious Diseases

Summary

Infectious diseases are caused by bacteria, viruses, fungi, and parasites. Infectious diseases are promoted by low socioeconomic status, poor hygiene, poor nutritional status, surgical procedures, poor tissue perfusion, long hospital stays, cancer, use of cytostatics, use of glucocorticoids, and use of antibiotics without proper indication. Before drugs are used to treat infectious diseases, an accurate diagnosis must be made. The decisive factor in treatment of infectious diseases is elimination of disease-promoting factors. Several viral diseases and some bacterial diseases can be prevented by vaccination.

Memo

1. Elimination of disease-promoting factors is crucial in treatment of infectious diseases.
2. Diseases caused by bacteria are treated with antibacterial drugs (antibiotics).
3. Antibiotics should be used cautiously to avoid development of resistance.
4. Antibiotics can cause allergies, diarrhea, and fungal infections.
5. Certain diseases caused by viruses—including hepatitis C, human immunodeficiency virus (HIV), shingles, and herpes simplex—can be treated with virustatics.
6. For the new disease COVID-19 (coronavirus disease 2019), which is caused by SARS-CoV-2 (severe acute respiratory syndrome coronavirus 2), no universal drug is available as yet.
7. Fungal infections of the skin, hair, and nails can be treated with terbinafine.
8. Yeast infections can be treated with azole antimycotics.
9. For treatment of scabies caused by mites, permethrin and ivermectin are effective.
10. For treatment of head lice infestations, dimethicone and ivermectin are effective.

How Do Infectious Diseases Develop?

Infectious diseases are caused by pathogens. These include bacteria, viruses, fungi, and parasites. Figure 11.3 provides an overview of the development, prevention, and treatment of infectious diseases. Health-promoting factors include a good immune system, good nutritional status, good tissue perfusion, good hygiene, and high socioeconomic status. Social distancing and wearing mouth–nose protection contribute to prevention of infectious diseases.

Disease-promoting factors for infectious diseases include poor nutritional status and a poor immune system. The function of the immune system is impaired by many drugs that are used to treat cancer and autoimmune

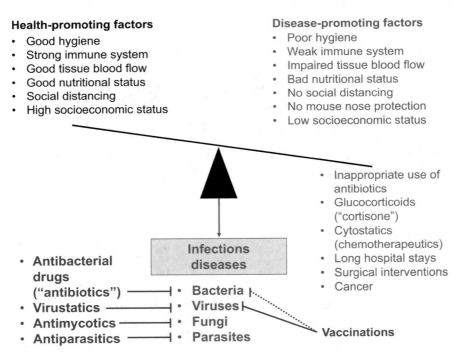

Fig. 11.3 How do infectious diseases develop, and how are they treated? Many infectious diseases are caused by dominance of disease-promoting factors as opposed to health-promoting factors. Infectious diseases are caused by bacteria, viruses, fungi, or parasites. The term "antibiotics" is misleading because it suggests that these drugs are effective against all pathogens. These drugs act only against bacteria, which is why they should be called antibacterial drugs. Inappropriate use of antibiotics is a major reason why bacteria are becoming resistant to many antibacterial drugs. Use of glucocorticoids (see Sect. 11.2) and cytostatics (see Sect. 11.1) promotes infectious diseases. Vaccinations can prevent infectious diseases, especially those caused by viruses

diseases (see Sects. 11.1 and 11.2). Long hospital stays and surgical interventions favor development of infectious diseases, as does poor tissue perfusion (e.g., after injuries or in diabetes; see Sect. 6.1). Other factors that promote infectious diseases are poor hygiene, close social contact, and low socioeconomic status. In some cases, especially in diseases caused by bacteria and fungi, the pathogens are not carried into the body from the outside; rather, they are a normal component of the microbiome. Microorganisms from the microbiome become pathogens under unfavorable conditions. Urinary tract infections, respiratory tract infections, and skin infections are often caused by bacteria from the microbiome, as are skin fungal and yeast infections.

Vaccinations

Vaccinations are effective measures to prevent infectious diseases. Effective and well-tolerated vaccines are available for diphtheria, whooping cough, measles, mumps, rubella, and smallpox. Vaccinations against influenza and COVID-19 are effective but must be repeated because the viruses continue to change genetically.

No Therapy Without a Proper Diagnosis

Before an infectious disease is treated, a precise diagnosis must be made. The pathogens causing the disease should be detected using suitable methods (e.g., detection of rod bacteria in urine in the case of urinary tract infection, viral genes in the case of COVID-19, yeasts in the case of candidiasis, or nits on hair in the case of head lice infestation). Sometimes the doctor is guided by clinical symptoms (e.g., urinary urgency and a burning sensation in the case of urinary tract infection; whitish deposits on the skin in the case of candidiasis; fever, shortness of breath, and taste disorders in the case of COVID-19; and itching of the scalp in the case of head lice). A reasonable compromise between the diagnostic effort and the severity of the disease must be reached. As a rule, the more severe a disease is, the greater the diagnostic effort must be.

Antibiotics: A Misleading Term

No universal drug for the treatment of infectious diseases exists. The term "antibiotics" (derived from the Greek word *bios*, meaning "life") suggests these drugs are effective against all pathogens of infectious diseases. However, this misconception only encourages misuse of these drugs and enhances the resistance problem (see section "Use Antibiotics Wisely"). The drugs known as "antibiotics" are actually antibacterial drugs. Within this class of drugs, large differences exist as to which drug is effective against which bacteria. Therefore, no antibacterial drug should be taken unless it is prescribed by a doctor. Antibiotics do not have an antipyretic effect. Unlike human cells, bacteria possess a cell wall that protects them from environmental influences. Therefore, inhibition of cell wall formation is an important target for antibiotics.

Use Antibiotics Wisely

Antibiotics are often prescribed without confirmation as to whether a bacterial infection is present. The use of "broad-spectrum antibiotics" is problematic. It is not clear which drugs constitute broad-spectrum antibiotics and which pathogens are targeted. Large-scale use of antibiotics in factory farming and insufficient hospital hygiene contribute significantly to development of antibiotic resistance. Uncritical use of broad-spectrum antibiotics promotes development of bacteria that are resistant to numerous antibacterial drugs. Multidrug-resistant *Staphylococcus aureus* (MRSA) can cause life-threatening hospital infections.

As a patient, you can help to ensure that antibiotics are used sparingly. Do not urge your doctor to prescribe an antibiotic "just in case". Another contribution you can make is to never take leftover antibiotics from a previous treatment without consulting a doctor. Fever, weakness, and coughing are not a sufficient reason to take antibiotics. Moreover, as a consumer, simply do not buy cheap poultry or pork produced by factory farming.

Antibiotic Treatment and Adverse Drug Reactions

The duration of treatment with antibiotics varies depending on the pathogen. Uncomplicated urinary tract infections in women can be treated with a single dose of fosfomycin. The typical treatment duration for a respiratory tract infection is 5 days, and that for Lyme disease is 2–3 weeks. Tuberculosis is treated for 6 months with several drugs in combination to prevent development of resistance. Antibiotics disrupt the gastrointestinal microbiome. This can result in diarrhea (see Sect. 3.3) or fungal infections (see section "Fungal Infections"). In the case of mild diarrhea, antibiotic therapy can usually be continued. In more severe diarrhea (pseudomembranous enterocolitis), the antibiotic must be discontinued. Clindamycin is an antibiotic with a high risk of causing pseudomembranous enterocolitis, so it should be used only with caution. Pseudomembranous enterocolitis is treated with metronidazole (see Sect. 3.2).

Antibiotics can cause allergies. Sulfonamides pose the greatest allergy risk (see Sect. 4.1). Sulfonamides are one component of cotrimoxazole, which is frequently used for urinary tract infections. Because of the allergy risk, cotrimoxazole should be used only if no alternative is available. Penicillins and cephalosporins (which are both beta-lactam antibiotics) pose an allergy risk, especially when applied locally on mucous membranes.

Beta-Lactam Antibiotics

Two of the most used beta-lactam antibiotics are amoxicillin and cefuroxime. They are effective against several bacterial pathogens causing respiratory or urinary tract infections. It is best to use these two antibiotics only if sensitivity of the pathogen has been demonstrated by an antibiogram. This will largely prevent development of resistance. The most common ADRs caused by amoxicillin and cefuroxime are diarrhea (see Sect. 3.3) and allergy (see Sect. 4.1). Many patients claim that they have a "penicillin allergy", although this is not the case. If there is any doubt, allergy testing should be performed. Use of beta-lactam antibiotics during pregnancy is not problematic.

Macrolides

If beta-lactam antibiotics cannot be used because they are not effective or because of ADRs, there are several alternatives. The macrolide antibiotic azithromycin is often used. This antibiotic is usually well tolerated. One disadvantage (in comparison with beta-lactam antibiotics) is that macrolide antibiotics do not kill bacteria; they only inhibit their growth. Thus, when a patient is treated with azithromycin, their immune system must work harder to overcome the infection. For this reason, beta-lactam antibiotics are preferred for use in immunocompromised patients, especially patients being treated for cancer or autoimmune disease (see Sects. 11.1 and 11.2). Macrolide antibiotics may be used during pregnancy.

Fluoroquinolones

Ciprofloxacin, from the class of fluoroquinolones, is another commonly used antibiotic. The duration of treatment with fluoroquinolones (the international nonproprietary names [INNs] of all drugs in this class have the characteristic suffix "_floxacin") should not exceed 2 weeks. Ciprofloxacin can cause tendon ruptures (especially rupture of the Achilles tendon). In addition, ciprofloxacin can cause confusion, hallucinations, and seizures. Therefore, caution should be exercised when this drug is used in patients with mental disorders (see Sects. 9.1–9.4). Ciprofloxacin should not be taken with calcium or dairy products, as calcium inhibits absorption of the antibiotic into the body (see Sect. 1.5).

Tetracyclines

The tetracycline doxycycline is a widely used antibiotic. Like ciprofloxacin, doxycycline should not be taken with calcium or dairy products, otherwise the drug will not be absorbed into the body (see Sect. 1.5). Doxycycline can cause skin hypersensitivity to UV radiation. It is therefore important that the patient avoids excessive sun exposure, uses sunblock, and covers the skin with clothing. Doxycycline must not be used during pregnancy, because the drug can be deposited in the teeth of the fetus and cause permanent yellowish discoloration.

How Are Viral Infectious Diseases Treated?

Viruses that affect humans need (human) host cells in order to reproduce. A basic distinction is made between DNA (deoxyribonucleic acid) viruses and RNA (ribonucleic acid) viruses. Highly effective and well-tolerated vaccines against some viral diseases (e.g., measles, mumps, rubella, and smallpox) are available.

Hepatitis C and HIV infection are examples of viral diseases that can be treated with a combination of different drugs. Hepatitis C must be treated for several months. HIV infection requires lifelong treatment because it is a retrovirus, meaning that the genetic material of the virus becomes incorporated into human DNA. Treatment of hepatitis C and HIV infection is carried out in special clinics. A detailed discussion of these treatments is beyond the scope of this book. An important pharmacoeconomic problem in treatment of hepatitis C and HIV infection are the high treatment costs.

The hepatitis C virus, the Ebola virus, and the SARS-CoV-2 coronavirus (which causes COVID-19) are RNA viruses. An important treatment strategy is therefore to inhibit RNA polymerase, which is important for replication of the genetic material of these viruses. Effective RNA polymerase inhibitors for hepatitis C (e.g., ledipasvir and simeprevir) are on the market.

The "Ebola drug" remdesivir has been repurposed and approved for COVID-19. Remdesivir shortens the course of severe forms of COVID-19. Several effective vaccines against SARS-CoV-2 have been approved. Systematic vaccination of the population in all countries of the world represents the only realistic possibility of getting the pandemic under control as soon as possible and returning to a "normal" life. Claims that RNA-based vaccines can cause genetic changes in the human genome are false. RNA cannot be transcribed into DNA by human enzymes; thus, it cannot be incorporated into human DNA. RNA is degraded rapidly in the body.

Influenza

The influenza virus is an RNA virus. Influenza vaccines are available, but the genes of the virus genome mutate quickly, which makes development of vaccines difficult. One can only make an educated guess as to which form of the virus will be most active in the next season, and then develop an appropriate vaccine. Just how effective the resulting vaccine will be depends on how good or bad a guess has been made. For example, the influenza vaccine is much less effective than the polio vaccine or the rubella vaccine.

Oseltamivir inhibits viral spread in the body but is clinically ineffective. Annual vaccination is crucial in the fight against influenza, especially in high-risk groups (elderly people, health professionals, and patients with chronic lung disease). In the case of influenza, bed rest and symptomatic therapy with analgesics and antipyretic drugs (see Sect. 2.1) are important, as is adequate fluid intake.

Herpes Infections

The chickenpox virus (varicella zoster virus) belongs to the DNA viruses. After varicella infection, the virus persists in the nerves responsible for perception of touch, temperature, and pain (sensory nerves). Various triggers (e.g.,

UV light, stress, cancer, or administration of cytostatics; see Sect. 11.1) can lead to reactivation of the infection (herpes zoster). It initially manifests itself in burning pain along the nerve fibers. A typical site of manifestation of herpes zoster is the nerve fibers along the ribs. The pain radiates from the spine to the sternum. Later, vesicles form and are scabbed over. Herpes zoster can vary in severity, from mild to life threatening. Timely diagnosis of herpes zoster is crucial. It is best to start treatment as soon as the typical burning pain appears, but at the latest, it should be started when the first blisters appear.

The drug of choice for herpes zoster is aciclovir, which inhibits DNA polymerase and thus inhibits replication of the virus genome. In mild courses, a 5- to 7-day treatment with oral aciclovir is sufficient. In severe cases, treatment with intravenous aciclovir is required. Aciclovir is well tolerated. Adequate fluid intake is crucial. Aciclovir is excreted by the kidneys, and insufficient fluid intake may lead to formation of aciclovir stones in the urinary tract.

Herpes simplex virus is another DNA virus, which can cause burning blisters in the mouth or the genital area. Local treatment with aciclovir ointments is usually sufficient. Timely diagnosis and early commencement of treatment are decisive.

Fungal Infections

Fungi are classified into dermatophytes (skin fungi), yeasts, and molds. Dermatophytes and yeasts are components of the microbiome of the human body. Normally, dermatophytes and yeasts don't cause diseases. Development of fungal diseases is favored by poor or exaggerated hygiene, heavy sweating, visits to public saunas or swimming pools, administration of antibiotics or glucocorticoids (see Sect. 11.2), and old age. Molds are present in moist potting soil and in the walls of damp dwellings, and they can cause serious systemic disease (aspergillosis). However, infections with dermatophytes and yeasts are much more common.

Dermatophyte Infections

Skin fungi can infect skin, hair, and nails. Typical symptoms are redness, itching, and oozing of the skin. Nail fungus is characterized by nail discoloration and brittleness. Fungal infestation of the scalp leads to hair loss. The fungi are detected microscopically. Depending on the severity and localization, systemic (oral) or local treatment is used. The most important drug for treatment of fungal skin infections is terbinafine. It inhibits formation of fungal cell membranes. This causes fungal cells to develop holes (pores), ultimately leading to the death of the cells. Terbinafine is generally well tolerated. However, after local administration, an allergic reaction can develop. With systemic administration, gastrointestinal problems (nausea, constipation, and diarrhea) or headaches can occur. Elimination of factors that favor fungal infection and adherence to good body hygiene are crucial for long-term success of skin fungus treatment with terbinafine.

Yeast Infections

The most important yeast fungus is *Candida albicans.* This fungus can cause local disease (local candidosis) or systemic candidosis (e.g., during treatment with cytostatics; see Sect. 11.1). Local candidosis is common. It is characterized by whitish coatings on mucous membranes, and the mucous membranes are often reddened and itchy. Typical sites of manifestation are the mouth (oral candidosis) and the genital area of women (vulvovaginal mycosis). A warm, moist environment favors candidosis, as does use of glucocorticoids (see Sects. 4.1 and 11.2) or antibiotics (which alters the microbiome). Similarly, patients with diabetes are at increased risk of candidosis (see Sect. 6.1). Therapy with gliflozins leads to greater excretion of sugar (glucose) in the urine. The yeast cells use this sugar as a nutrient, and this can promote development of candidosis in the genital area by overgrowing the microbiome (see Sect. 6.1).

Yeast infections can be treated effectively with antimycotics whose INNs have the suffix "_azole". Azoles destroy the structure of the fungal cell membrane. This causes the fungal cells to become holey, which finally leads to their death. Azole antimycotics can be used locally and systemically. In uncomplicated courses of candidosis in the intimate area, a 1-day treatment with an azole antimycotic (clotrimazole) is sufficient. The drug is applied as vaginal suppository and a cream. It is crucial to eliminate any factors that facilitate infection. Soaps, body washes, and cleansers should not come into direct contact with the vagina, and it is recommended to wear breathable underwear and avoid tight pants.

Parasite Infections

Scabies (caused by mites) and head lice are common parasite diseases. Both diseases occur particularly in kindergartens, schools, large families, and collective accommodation—i.e., in situations where close social contact and transmission of pathogens from one person to another are favored.

Scabies is characterized by reddish mite ducts in the skin and severe itching. The wandering mites can be seen in the ducts. Treatment is simple and effective. Oral (systemic) treatment with ivermectin or local treatment with permethrin can be used. These two drugs act on the nervous system of the mites, killing them. Ivermectin is well tolerated. With permethrin, skin burning may occur. For scabies prophylaxis, good hygiene in facilities (as well as in the household) and avoidance of close body contact are necessary.

Head lice infestation is characterized by itching. The diagnosis is made by detection of sticky, elongated nits on the hair. To get rid of lice, ivermectin or dimethicone is applied to the hair, and the hair is then combed. Ivermectin paralyzes the nervous system of the lice; dimethicone destroys the carapace of the lice. These drugs are well tolerated. Treatment of the entire family in which a head lice infestation has occurred is strongly recommended. To prevent head lice infestations in groups, avoid close contact and adhere to hygiene measures. Combs and brushes should never be shared by different people.

Glossary of Important Pharmacological Terms

Commonly used term (frequently used synonyms are written in parentheses)	Explanation (the correct term, if available, is shown in bold text)	Examples (drug-specific syllables [or word stems] are shown in bold text)
Active substance (pharmacologically active substance)	Any chemical substance that affects bodily functions. Includes drugs and poisons. The term says nothing about usefulness or harmfulness	
Adherence (compliance)	The term describes the patient's willingness to regularly take the medicine prescribed for them by a doctor. In the past, adherence was often enforced by authoritarian doctors, with correspondingly low success. The key to high adherence and thus to successful therapy is that the patient understands why they have to take a drug and what positive effects and adverse reactions they can expect from the therapy	

(continued)

(continued)

Commonly used term (frequently used synonyms are written in parentheses)	Explanation (the correct term, if available, is shown in bold text)	Examples (drug-specific syllables [or word stems] are shown in bold text)
Adverse drug effect (adverse drug reaction, ADR, side effect)	In many cases, an adverse drug reaction can be derived from the mechanism of action of a drug. For some drug classes, drug allergy plays a role	
Agonist (_mimetic)	A drug that activates a receptor and thereby mimics the effects of a first messenger (hormone, neurotransmitter, mediator of inflammation)	Serotonin-1 receptor agonists (triptans), beta sympathomimetics, incretin mimetics
Aldosterone antagonists	**Mineralocorticoid receptor antagonists** (MCRAs). These drugs not only inhibit the effect of aldosterone but also inhibit the effect of cortisol	Spironolactone, eplerenone (ten times more expensive than spironolactone)
Antagonist (blocker, anti_, _lytic)	A drug that binds to a receptor but does not activate it. By binding to the receptor, the antagonist prevents activation of the receptor by a first messenger (hormone, neurotransmitter, mediator of inflammation)	Serotonin-3 receptor antagonists (setrons), beta blockers (beta receptor antagonists), antihistamines (H_1 receptor antagonists), parasympatholytics (muscarinic receptor antagonists)
Anti_	The syllable "anti" means that a drug class has an effect against a particular disease (or symptom). The term originates from a time when the mechanisms of action of drugs were not yet understood. "Anti_" is part of a generic term that covers drug classes with very different mechanisms. In the meantime, the fields of application of many "anti_" drugs have expanded. This often leads to confusion among patients and doctors. It is generally better to refer to "**drugs with an anti_ effect**". This description is more cumbersome but allows for the possibility that the drug in question also has other effects	Antiallergics, antiarrhythmics, antibiotics, anticholinergics, antidepressants, antidiabetics, antiemetics, antihypertensives, antiepileptics, antihistamines, antipsychotics

(continued)

(continued)

Commonly used term (frequently used synonyms are written in parentheses)	Explanation (the correct term, if available, is shown in bold text)	Examples (drug-specific syllables [or word stems] are shown in bold text)
Antiarrhythmics	Problematic term because many antiarrhythmic drugs can also cause cardiac arrhythmias (i.e., they have a proarrhythmic effect). This is easily overlooked when the term "antiarrhythmics" is used. It is better to speak of "drugs with an antiarrhythmic effect"	Amiodarone (a drug that blocks numerous ion channels) is the gold standard of antiarrhythmics although it can cause adverse drug reactions
Antibiotics	**Antibacterial drugs.** Contrary to what the term suggests (*bios* is Greek for "life"), "antibiotics" are not effective against viruses and fungi. The imprecise term "antibiotics" promotes use of antibacterial drugs without proper indication. They are prescribed far too often	Amoxicillin, clarithromycin, moxifloxacin, doxycycline
Antidepressants	**Generic term for very different drugs with antidepressant effects.** Since these drugs are also used for many other neurological and mental disorders, it is better to use the names of the individual drug classes and to avoid use of the term "antidepressants". The term "depression" evokes negative associations. Patients who are prescribed "antidepressants" (for another condition) probably will not take these drugs regularly because they assume that they are depressed	Amitriptyline (a nonselective monoamine reuptake inhibitor), citalopram (a selective serotonin reuptake inhibitor), venlafaxine (a selective serotonin/norepinephrine reuptake inhibitor), alpha-2 receptor antagonists (mirtazapine), monoamine oxidase inhibitors (tranylcypromine). A common feature of all these drugs is that they enhance the effects of the neurotransmitters norepinephrine and/or serotonin. Most therapeutic effects and adverse drug reactions can be explained by these mechanisms

(*continued*)

(continued)

Commonly used term (frequently used synonyms are written in parentheses)	Explanation (the correct term, if available, is shown in bold text)	Examples (drug-specific syllables [or word stems] are shown in bold text)
Antiepileptics (anticonvulsants)	**Generic term for very different drugs with antiepileptic effects.** As these drugs are also used to treat many other neurological and psychiatric diseases, the term "antiepileptics" should be replaced by the specific name of the drug class or drug	Pregabalin (a calcium channel blocker); carbamazepine, lamotrigine, phenytoin, valproic acid (sodium channel blockers)
Antihistamines	**Histamine H$_1$ receptor antagonists (H$_1$ receptor antagonists)**	Clemastine (easily crosses the blood–brain barrier), cetirizine (a second-generation antihistamine, which crosses the blood–brain barrier less easily)
Antihypertensives (blood pressure drugs)	**Generic term for very different drugs with antihypertensive (blood pressure–lowering) effects.** Since some of these drugs are also used for other cardiovascular diseases such as coronary heart disease and chronic heart failure (especially drug classes A, B, and D), the term "antihypertensives" should be replaced by the specific name of the drug class or drug	Drug classes A, B, C, and D
Antipsychotics (neuroleptics)	**Generic term for very different drugs with antipsychotic effects.** Since these drugs are used not only for schizophrenia but also for other neurological and mental diseases, the term "antipsychotics" should be replaced by the name of the specific drug class or drug. "Neuroleptics" is an obsolete term	A common feature of all of these drugs is that they act as antagonists at many (multiple) receptors. Classification of antipsychotics into "typical" and "atypical" antipsychotics is no longer reasonable and is obsolete

(continued)

(continued)

Commonly used term (frequently used synonyms are written in parentheses)	Explanation (the correct term, if available, is shown in bold text)	Examples (drug-specific syllables [or word stems] are shown in bold text)
Aspirin-induced asthma	**Cyclooxygenase (COX) inhibitor-induced asthma.** This type of asthma occurs not only with acetylsalicylic acid but also with other COX inhibitors such as ibuprofen and diclofenac. It does not occur with paracetamol or metamizole	
Beta blockers	**Beta receptor antagonists.** Usually, only beta-1 receptor antagonists are meant. Therefore, it is better to use the exact drug class name	Propran**olol** (a nonselective beta receptor antagonist), metop**rolol** (a selective **beta-1** receptor antagonist)
Beta sympathomimetics	**Beta receptor agonists.** Almost always, only beta-2 receptor agonists are meant. Therefore, it is better to use the exact drug class name	**Beta-2** receptor agonists: albut**erol** (a short-acting beta receptor antagonist [SABA]), form**oterol** (a long-acting beta receptor antagonist [LABA])
Blood clotting inhibitors (anticoagulants)	**Generic term for two drug classes:** factor Xa inhibitors and vitamin K antagonists (coumarins)	Factor Xa inhibitors: rivar**oxa**ban; vitamin K antagonists: warfarin
Broad-spectrum antibiotics	**Problematic generic term.** It is not clearly defined which "antibiotics" (antibacterial drugs) are included. Moreover, resistance of bacteria can change rapidly, both locally and over time. The term "broad-spectrum" also suggests a false sense of security	Aminopenicillins, macrolides, fluoroquinolones, tetracyclines

(continued)

(continued)

Commonly used term (frequently used synonyms are written in parentheses)	Explanation (the correct term, if available, is shown in bold text)	Examples (drug-specific syllables [or word stems] are shown in bold text)
Cardiac glycosides (digitalis glycosides)	**Sodium/potassium ATPase inhibitors.** The term "cardiac glycosides" suggests a selective and positive effect on the heart, which is not the case at all. Cardiac glycosides act in every cell of the body because the target (sodium/potassium ATPase) is present in every cell. This is why cardiac glycosides cause so many adverse drug reactions and why treatment with these drugs is so difficult to control, despite therapeutic drug monitoring. The term "digitalis glycosides" is better because it refers to the plant the drugs are made of (foxglove, *Digitalis purpurea*)	**Dig**oxin
Chemotherapy ("chemo")	**Treatment of a malignant disease (cancer therapy) with cytostatics.** Actually, treatment with antibacterial drugs, virostatics, and antifungals is also chemotherapy. However, the term "chemotherapy" is commonly used for treatment of cancer	Cyclophosphamide, methotrexate, paclitaxel
Cholesterol reducers (statins, lipid-lowering drugs)	**HMG-CoA reductase inhibitors.** The term "cholesterol reducers" has a positive connotation and often causes the doctor and patient to forget that these drugs can also cause severe adverse drug reactions in muscles. There are also other "cholesterol reducers" (e.g., fibrates)	Simva**statin**

(continued)

(continued)

Commonly used term (frequently used synonyms are written in parentheses)	Explanation (the correct term, if available, is shown in bold text)	Examples (drug-specific syllables [or word stems] are shown in bold text)
Cortisone (steroids, corticosteroids, cortisone derivatives)	**Glucocorticoids (glucocorticoid receptor agonists).** The hormone cortisol (commonly called "cortisone") is the most important endogenous glucocorticoid and is practically only used in adrenal cortical failure (Addison's disease) as a substitute (supplementation) for the missing hormone. "Steroids" is a generic term that also includes mineralocorticoids (e.g., aldosterone) and sex hormones (estrogen, progesterone, testosterone)	Prednisolone, budesonide
Direct oral anticoagulants (DOACs) or new oral anticoagulants (NOACs)	**Factor Xa inhibitors.** The terms "direct" or "new" suggest advantages over vitamin K antagonists, but that is not correct. Moreover, factor Xa inhibitors are not "new"; they have been around since the early 2000s	Riva**roxaban**
Diuretics (strong)	**Inhibitors of the sodium/ potassium/chloride cotransporter, NKCC inhibitors** ("loop diuretics"). These diuretics also cause clinically important vasodilation. The term "diuretics" focuses too much on the diuretic effect	Furo**semide**
Diuretics (weak)	**Inhibitors of the sodium/ chloride cotransporter, NCC inhibitors** ("thiazide diuretics"). These diuretics also cause clinically important vasodilation. The term "diuretics" focuses too much on the diuretic effect	Chlorthalidone

(continued)

(continued)

Commonly used term (frequently used synonyms are written in parentheses)	Explanation (the correct term, if available, is shown in bold text)	Examples (drug-specific syllables [or word stems] are shown in bold text)
Drug class A	**Renin–angiotensin–aldosterone system inhibitors (RAAS inhibitors).** This class comprises angiotensin-converting enzyme inhibitors (ACE inhibitors) and angiotensin receptor antagonists (angiotensin receptor blockers [ARBs]). This drug class has antihypertensive effects and also prevents connective tissue remodeling processes in the heart that occur in heart attacks and heart failure	Rami**pril**, cande**sartan**
Drug class B (beta blockers)	**Beta-1 receptor antagonists.** This drug class has antihypertensive effects and protects the heart from dangerous overactivation by the sympathetic nervous system in heart attacks (coronary heart disease) and heart failure. In addition, drug class B can reduce the heart rate in atrial fibrillation	Metop**rolol**
Drug class C (calcium antagonists)	**Calcium channel blockers.** This drug class mainly has antihypertensive effects	Amlo**dipine**
Drug class D (diuretics)	**Inhibitors of the sodium–chloride cotransporter** ("thiazide diuretics") and **inhibitors of sodium–potassium–chloride cotransporters** ("loop diuretics"). In hypertension, the main focus is on the blood pressure–lowering effect. In heart failure, the diuretic effect of this drug class is in the foreground	Furo**semide**

(continued)

(continued)

Commonly used term (frequently used synonyms are written in parentheses)	Explanation (the correct term, if available, is shown in bold text)	Examples (drug-specific syllables [or word stems] are shown in bold text)
Epinephrine (EPI, adrenaline, stress hormone)	**Epinephrine** generally has a bad reputation as a harmful stress hormone. While it is true that continuous release of epinephrine can lead to cardiovascular diseases, a single administration of epinephrine is life saving in life-threatening allergic (anaphylactic) shock. Epinephrine anxiety is widespread among doctors, leading to infrequent use of epinephrine in allergic emergencies and resulting in unnecessary deaths of patients	Patients with a severe allergy should always carry an epinephrine auto-injector (or preferably two) with them—epinephrine for self-treatment!
Gliflozins	**Inhibitors of renal glucose reabsorption (SGLT-2 inhibitors)**	Empa**gliflozin**
Gliptins	**Incretin enhancer** (inhibitors of incretin degradation, DPP-4 inhibitors, dipeptidyl peptidase-4 inhibitors)	Sita**gliptin**
H_2 receptor blockers	**Histamine H_2 receptor antagonists (H_2 receptor antagonists).** Not to be confused with antihistamines (histamine H_1 receptor antagonists, H_1 receptor antagonists). Both drug classes are histamine receptor antagonists but act at different receptors	Rani**tidine**

(continued)

(continued)

Commonly used term (frequently used synonyms are written in parentheses)	Explanation (the correct term, if available, is shown in bold text)	Examples (drug-specific syllables [or word stems] are shown in bold text)
Hormones	It is a widespread assumption that hormones are harmful. This misconception applies in particular to glucocorticoids (cortisone) and sex hormones (estrogen, gestagen). Sex hormones in particular have a bad reputation when applied during menopause, which is why women turn to herbal preparations that supposedly work better and are safer. Actually, the supply of hormones (e.g., in the case of hypothyroidism or adrenal cortical hypofunction) can be life saving. In many cases, treatment is carried out not with hormones but with drugs derived from hormones	Hormones: levothyroxine, estrogen, gestagen, cortisol, testosterone, aldosterone Hormone derivatives: drugs in contraceptives (morning-after pill, mini-pill, micro-pill), prednisolone (treatment of autoimmune diseases), budesonide (treatment of asthma and ulcerative colitis)
Incretin mimetics	**Incretin receptor agonists**	Liraglutide
Mood stabilizers (phase prophylaxis)	**Generic term** for very different drugs that can balance the mood in bipolar disorder and depression. Since these drugs also have other effects (e.g., valproic acid and lamotrigine have an antiepileptic effect), it is better not to use the term "mood stabilizers" but to instead use the term **"drugs with a mood-stabilizing effect"**	Lithium, valproic acid, lamotrigine
Nonopioid analgesics	**Generic term** for cyclooxygenase-2 inhibitors and other analgesics such as paracetamol (acetaminophen) and metamizole (dipyrone). Nonopioid analgesics do not have a common mechanism of action	Ibuprofen, diclofenac, etori**coxib**, paracetamol, metamizole

(continued)

(continued)

Commonly used term (frequently used synonyms are written in parentheses)	Explanation (the correct term, if available, is shown in bold text)	Examples (drug-specific syllables [or word stems] are shown in bold text)
Nonsteroidal anti-inflammatory drugs (NSAIDs)	(Nonselective) **cyclooxygenase inhibitors (COX inhibitors).** Sometimes metamizole (dipyrone) and paracetamol are erroneously assigned to the NSAIDs, although they have very different therapeutic effects and adverse drug reactions	Ibu**profen**, diclofen**ac**
Opioid analgesics (morphine, opium, opioids, opiates)	**Opioid receptor agonists.** This term is more appropriate because this drug class has many other clinically useful effects (and many adverse drug reactions) in addition to its analgesic effect. The term "opioids" is derived from the fact that the first analgesics of this drug class were derived from opium (obtained from opium poppies). Opioid analgesic addiction is commonly referred to as heroin addiction because heroin has such a strong and rapid effect. However, fentanyl now plays a more important role in addiction than heroin	Morphine and fentanyl (highly effective), buprenorphine (moderately effective), tramadol (weakly effective). Loperamide (for treatment of diarrhea) is also an opioid receptor agonist
Oral antidiabetics	**Generic term** for very different classes of orally administered drugs for treatment of type 2 diabetes. Since the efficacy and adverse drug reactions of the individual drug classes vary substantially and some of these classes are also used for other diseases, it is better not to use the term "oral antidiabetics" but to use the name of the respective drug class instead	Metformin (biguanides), glibenclamide (sulfonylureas), empa**gliflozin** (gliflozins), sita**gliptin** (gliptins), pio**glitazone** (glitazones)

(continued)

(continued)

Commonly used term (frequently used synonyms are written in parentheses)	Explanation (the correct term, if available, is shown in bold text)	Examples (drug-specific syllables [or word stems] are shown in bold text)
Parasympatholytics (anticholinergics, antimuscarinics)	**Muscarinic receptor antagonists.** These drugs cause an anticholinergic (more correctly: antimuscarinic) syndrome: dry mouth, heartburn, palpitations, blurred vision, dry skin, constipation, and urinary retention are key symptoms	Biperiden, scopolamine, tiotropium (a long-acting muscarinic receptor antagonist), ipratropium (a short-acting muscarinic receptor antagonist), and many antihistamines, antipsychotics, and antidepressants have parasympatholytic effects
Platelet inhibitors (thrombocyte aggregation inhibitors, platelet aggregation inhibitors)	**Generic term for two drug classes:** irreversible cyclooxygenase inhibitors and adenosine diphosphate receptor antagonists	Irreversible cyclooxygenase inhibitors: acetylsalicylic acid (ASA); irreversible adenosine diphosphate receptor antagonists: clopido**grel**
Poison	A substance with a harmful effect on the body. Some poisons become drugs through targeted use, and drugs become poisons through overdose	Botulinum neurotoxin (poison if taken orally; drug if administered locally in muscles); paracetamol (pain relieving in doses of up to 4 grams per day, liver toxic in doses exceeding 8 grams per day)
Psychotropic drugs	**Generic term** for very different drug classes that have effects on the brain. Benzodiazepines and dopamimetics can cause addiction; antidepressants, antipsychotics, and mood stabilizers do not have these effects. It is therefore better to use the individual drug class names. Antiepileptic drugs also have important psychotropic effects but are not usually classified as "psychotropic drugs". The term "psychotropic drugs" has a negative connotation and is automatically associated with the potention for addiction, but this is incorrect	Antidepressants, antiepileptics, antipsychotics, benzodiazepines, dopamimetics, mood stabilizers

(continued)

(continued)

Commonly used term (frequently used synonyms are written in parentheses)	Explanation (the correct term, if available, is shown in bold text)	Examples (drug-specific syllables [or word stems] are shown in bold text)
Receptor	Sensor for first messengers (hormones, neurotransmitters, mediators of inflammation) in the body. Receptors are targets for agonists and antagonists	Beta receptors, dopamine receptors, histamine receptors, muscarinic receptors, serotonin receptors
Sartans (angiotensin receptor blockers, ARBs)	**Angiotensin receptor antagonists**	Cande**sartan**
Setrons	**Serotonin-3 receptor antagonists**	Ondan**setron**
Stomach protection	**Prophylaxis for heartburn and gastric/duodenal ulcers.** Routine administration of proton pump inhibitors in hospital/intensive care units or to patients treated with platelet aggregation inhibitors (especially acetylsalicylic acid) as prophylaxis for myocardial infarction or strokes. Prophylaxis with proton pump inhibitors should be critically evaluated. In the long term, proton pump inhibitors can cause severe adverse drug reactions	Pantoprazole
Sugar	**Informal term.** "Sugar" is often used to trivialize diabetes. There are very many different "sugars" (monosaccharides, disaccharides, and polymers such as the carbohydrate glycogen, which is stored in the liver). In the context of diabetes, the monosaccharide glucose (dextrose) is particularly relevant. In hypoglycemia (low blood sugar), other "sugars" such as sucrose do not have as rapid an effect as glucose	Glucose

(*continued*)

(continued)

Commonly used term (frequently used synonyms are written in parentheses)	Explanation (the correct term, if available, is shown in bold text)	Examples (drug-specific syllables [or word stems] are shown in bold text)
Tricyclic antidepressants (tricyclics, TCAs)	**Nonselective monoamine reuptake inhibitors (NSMRIs).** The term "tricyclic antidepressants" refers to the chemical structure of these drugs	Ami**triptyline**
Triptans	**Serotonin-1 receptor agonists**	Suma**triptan**
Z drugs	Drugs (the prototype drug is zolpidem) with effects similar to those of benzodiazepines, only shorter and weaker	

Further Reading

1. Seifert R. *Basic Knowledge of Pharmacology*. Cham: Springer; 2019. (This is a short textbook on pharmacology—an adaptation of a German textbook titled *Basiswissen Pharmakologie*—for an international audience. It includes case reports and lists selected literature for further reading.)
2. Brunton LL, Hilal-Dandan R, Knollmann BJ (editors). *Goodman & Gilman's: The Pharmacological Basis of Therapeutics*. 13th edition. New York: McGraw-Hill; 2017. (This multiauthor book is a very comprehensive and detailed reference work with an extensive bibliography. It is well suited to in-depth study and focuses on the situation in the USA.)
3. Ritter J, Flower R, Henderson G, Loke YK, McEwan D, Rang H. *Rang & Dale's Pharmacology*. 9th edition. Amsterdam: Elsevier; 2019. (This comprehensive textbook on pharmacology covers basic pharmacology and clinical pharmacology. It focuses on the situation in Great Britain.)

Printed in the United States
by Baker & Taylor Publisher Services